Dancing
in Limbo

Dancing in Limbo

Making Sense of Life After Cancer

Glenna Halvorson-Boyd
Lisa K. Hunter

Jossey-Bass Publishers   San Francisco

Substantial discounts on bulk quantities of Jossey-Bass books are available to corporations, professional associations, and other organizations. For details and discount information, contact the special sales department at Jossey-Bass Inc., Publishers.(415) 433-1740; Fax (800) 605-2665.

For sales outside the United States, please contact your local Simon & Schuster International Office.

www.josseybass.com

 Manufactured in the United States of America on Lyons Falls Turin Book. This paper is acid-free and 100 percent totally chlorine-free.

Credits are on page 177.

Library of Congress Cataloging-in-Publication Data

Halvorson-Boyd, Glenna, date.
    Dancing in limbo : making sense of life after cancer / Glenna Halvorson-Boyd, Lisa K. Hunter.
       p.   cm.
    Includes bibliographical references.
    ISBN 0-7879-0103-2 (alk. paper)
    1. Cancer—Psychological aspects.   I. Hunter, Lisa. II. Title.
RC263.H27   1995
362.1'96994—dc20   95-9135

FIRST EDITION
HB Printing 10 9 8 7 6 5 4 3 2

To my father, Glenn Halvorson,
and my mother, Mary, and to my husband, Curtis.

To John and Skip, my family.

All these, upwhirled aloft,
Fly o'er the backside of the world far-off,
Into a limbo large and broad.
—Milton, *Paradise Lost*

Contents

1

Breaking the Silence

Limbo 1: A region on the border between hell and heaven where those who are not responsible for their fate await judgment day. These souls can neither be punished in purgatory nor received into heaven. They must simply wait.

Limbo 2: A state of being midway between two extremes.

Limbo 3: A dance of West Indian origin in which the dancer bends backward and shuffles under a horizontal bar that is lowered after each successive pass. The dance requires strength and flexibility.

ADAPTED FROM *WEBSTER'S THIRD NEW INTERNATIONAL DICTIONARY*

There is a cruel myth about surviving cancer. In this myth, when medical treatment is successful, the story ends. Having survived cancer, we pick up our lives where they were interrupted and carry on—with increased gratitude for the simple acts of daily life and the clarity of purpose that only a brush with death affords. In this myth, cancer is a blessing in disguise.

Though the myth has some truth, it is cruel because it is impossible to live. The real story does not end "happily ever after." Instead, we live in limbo: after cancer, we know that we are on uncertain ground.

1

In the beginning, we think that limbo is only as large as our cancer: Will I live or will I die from this disease? Then we get the lightening bolt. Limbo is the borderland where we will live for the rest of our lives. Although we cannot control our fate, we must do more than wait. We are responsible for how we live in whatever time we have, and whenever time is up, we will face our death again. That is the awesome, awful truth of limbo.

This book is the true story of our lives in limbo. We have both survived cancer. We have also struggled to make sense of the sad and frightening feelings that are omitted from the survival myth. When we resumed our daily lives, we were disoriented and confused. Everyone who had cared for us went on about his or her business, leaving us to ours. All the people we knew thought we were getting back to normal. Neither of us had realized that "normal" was gone.

We felt lost in the most familiar places—home and work and play—among the most familiar people—family and friends. Nothing seemed the same, and of course, it wasn't, because we were not the same. But the myth had worked its mischief: we felt crazy and alone. We were stuck in limbo, but we didn't know that yet. We had not begun to make sense of our lives after cancer.

Entering the Unknown

Very little is known about surviving cancer. There is a glut of information about diagnosis and treatment. Dozens of books give cancer patients advice: some tell us what to eat while others tell us what to think. A few beg our sympathy or hope to inspire us. Much of this is useful, but it is not what we need once our diagnosis and treatment are past. Why the silence about survival?

For years, no one would utter the C-word. Until the early 1970s, cancer patients were rarely told their diagnosis. This makes sense if we remember that the prospect of survival is relatively new. According to the American Cancer Society, in the early 1900s, few cancer patients had any hope of long-term survival. In the 1930s, fewer than one in five patients was alive five years after treatment. In the 1940s, it was one in four, and in the 1960s, it was one in three. This year, over a million Americans will be diagnosed with cancer, and nearly half will survive their disease. Today, there are more than eight million cancer survivors alive in the U.S., and their numbers are steadily increasing. It is time to talk about what it is really like to survive cancer.

The two of us decided to write the book that we could not find. The undertaking seemed straightforward at first, but breaking the silence proved tricky. As we wrote about death anxiety, our own resurfaced. We had to face the irrational fear that talking about survival would jinx our own cures. We also worried that if we told the truth, we would sound like ingrates: had we forgotten how lucky we are?

But when we talked with colleagues and friends about the book, our worries faded. They were interested, they wanted to understand, and they knew people we should talk to. That is how we found the other survivors you will meet in this book. To our surprise, everyone we asked agreed to an interview. Although most of the conversations began on a politely guarded note, everyone warmed to the topic. It was a relief to talk. The survivors spoke with candor, and we learned a lot. Yes, they are grateful to be alive. And, no, they aren't living happily ever after either. However, most of them believe that they are living more fully and authentically because they have faced death. And that confrontation is among the hardest work they have ever done.

We talked at length with five men and thirteen women. Their stories are woven throughout the book. They had different cancers at different stages of life. Their survival times range from seven months to thirty years. Although most of them are now in their forties and fifties, one was in her early twenties when she was first diagnosed and treated, another was in her mid seventies. In terms of age and type of cancer, they reflect national figures for cancer survival; however, they are not intended to be a representative sample of the U.S. population of cancer survivors. We spoke with more women than men, and all are white, well educated, and were able to afford treatment. We were seeking a range of experiences, and that was what we found. Despite these survivors' similarities, their stories are remarkably varied, and their experiences broadened and enriched our understanding of life after cancer. There are many more stories to be told, but the ones we tell help all of us understand more clearly what it means to be a cancer survivor.

This book is the record of a number of journeys through the nowhere land that we came to call limbo. It is a book for cancer survivors, their families and friends, and all the health care givers who work to save their lives. It began with our experiences and grew as we talked with other survivors. Although each experience is unique, the deeper issues are much the same. With cancer, people confront death. With survival, they feel an urgency to reexamine how they live the rest of their lives.

The Beginning of Our Stories

Ironically, our friendship began with cancer. We met years ago, in graduate school, but we didn't become close until our major professor was diagnosed with cancer. Within weeks, he was dead, and we turned to each other for support and sympathy. Years later, it felt natural for us to turn again to each other in the aftermath of our own cancers. We learned together that there was no right or easy way to re-create our lives after we had nearly lost them.

Glenna's Story

It has been more than ten years since I had a malignant tumor removed from the base of my tongue. Like many cancer survivors, I detected the sore and went promptly for care. When the dental hygienist said, "There's nothing there. You're just imagining things," I demanded my dentist. He probed with his long-necked mirror, and then, without a word, stripped off his gloves and threw them across the room. I closed my eyes and felt his hand gently touch my forearm. He simply said, "Oh god! I wish you weren't so smart," and I said, through my tears, "What do we do next?"

Within twenty-four hours, I had a diagnosis, and I had decided that cancer would not be a bad experience—as long as I survived. (I could change my mind later if the disease proved fatal.) I went to a medical school library and read all the diagnosis and treatment literature on oral cancer. After a harrowing day in the library, I recalled an old fear. In grammar school, one of my classmates had read my palm: "You have the shortest lifeline. You're going to die young." I remember running my fingernail along that line, trying to make it longer. That memory is recorded in my journal, on the page facing my notes from the *British Journal of Oral Surgery*. I wrote, as if in argument with that hateful little girl or to convince myself, "That line on my hand is not the length of my life. I am not going to die from this."

I had surgery one week before my thirty-seventh birthday. I told everyone what I wanted that year—to go home from the hospital without cancer. Although I'd stared too long at the awful pictures in the medical journals and was terrified that my face would be disfigured or that I would never speak, for the moment, that didn't matter. I just wanted to live, at any cost. I got my wish. When I left the hospital, I could not talk, but I had a hopeful prognosis and greater confidence in myself. I believed that my limits had been tested, and I had aced the test.

During the next year, so many bad things happened in my life that cancer seemed the least of my worries. There were deaths and accidents and business reversals. I felt an aching sense of defeat. I had wanted so desperately to live; now I was crying in my sleep. I didn't know what was happening.

Then, on a business trip to Jamaica, I had an insight. Although the setting was magnificent, the conference was long and dull. At one of the official dinners, there was a limbo contest. As the supple Jamaican dancers entertained the tourists, my mind wandered, and suddenly I was in tears. For me, limbo was not a dance; it was my life. My future was uncertain. No wonder I was crying.

Finally, I had a word for my vague misery. I took some comfort in the notion, but I didn't want to talk about it. I did not want to know that I had lost the invisible barrier between death and me. My mother and my grandmother had both survived breast cancer. They were my models of survival—and silence. They simply carried on, or so it had seemed to me, and I felt obliged to do the same.

Then my mother was rushed to the hospital in the night. She survived, but after a week, she left the hospital with a fatal diagnosis: massive radiation damage to her heart and lungs—a late effect of her cancer treatment. During the two and a half years that it took for her to die, all five of my aunts died. An entire generation of women disappeared from my life. It was too much: I had known death in my body. I took death personally.

Surviving cancer has been harder than I had expected. Living with terminal uncertainty is humbling, and I had underestimated its effect. Limbo was no longer a comforting abstraction; it was the ground falling away beneath me. Just then, my closest colleague died of pancreatic cancer, and three dear friends were diagnosed with cancer. Two were recurrences. One of them was Lisa.

Lisa's Story

I remember the night I learned that the lump under my arm was a tumor, the spread of my melanoma. I have always remembered my thoughts that night, but I have not wanted to revisit my feelings. Confronting impossible feelings is like being trapped in a box with very high sides. You run along the bottom looking for a crack of light or a hole that will lead you out of the box, but there isn't one. The box is reality: I have cancer in my body, and I can die from it. There is neither respite nor comfort—anywhere.

The night of the tumor diagnosis, I was alone. I talked with my brother and friends, and they comforted me on the phone, but no one could change the words on my answering machine: "Your biopsy was positive for tumor." My frantic mental scrabblings tried to erase them. In the night, each time I woke—heavy with anxiety in the pit of my stomach and, even half-conscious, knowing that something terrible was wrong—I willed myself back to sleep. Even in sleep, I dreamed, so there was no escape.

The thought I remember most clearly from that night was that I would be dead before I would be old enough to retire. I had just read Peter Mayle's book about retiring to Provence, and I wanted to see that French countryside, to eat and drink and walk in the warmth of the sun. I knew that night that I would never see Provence. Living long enough to retire was suddenly an impossible dream that I desperately wanted.

The next day and the days that followed, I walled off my feelings by taking action, organizing my information, my surgery, my work, my support. I had the clarity I had experienced when my mother died: the trivia of daily life drops away, and there is no question about what is important. This heady sense lasted through my leave of absence from work. There was order in the universe, and I was secure.

When I returned to work and "normal" life, I crashed. My work, my relationships, and my home were all the same, but I was different. I was worried, jumpy, forgetful, hopeless, and exhausted. I had always relied on my ability to organize things, but now everything seemed fragmented, disorganized, out of control. I was clinging to others and afraid of driving them away.

My clarity was gone, and my brain felt as if someone had melted cheese over it. I made a dim connection with what widows experience after the funeral is over, when friends drift away and they are left with the reality of loss.

I felt disoriented and depressed, and the worst part was not knowing why. My feelings didn't make sense. The crisis was over, and everything had turned out better than I had hoped. Why didn't I feel good? What was wrong with me?

I called Glenna. I don't remember what she said, only that when we stopped talking I knew that I wasn't crazy. I understood that I was beginning to cope with a trauma that had forever changed my life.

In the two years since that phone call, I have come a long way. I have been to Provence, moved to the country where I watch the birds and listen to the wind, formed an important love relationship, and dropped a burdensome job responsibility. I grit my teeth and acknowledge that I still have to work to keep my balance. I now assume that I have a future but try not to put off what's important to me. And I am planning for my retirement.

What's Different About Surviving Cancer?

Reflecting on our stories and those we heard from other cancer survivors raised an intriguing question: Why had surviving cancer thrown so many of us for a loop? As a group, we had ample experience with traumatic events. Most of us had lost at least one parent, several had been divorced, several were widowed, and several more had lost a child. We had had other serious illnesses and injuries and potentially fatal accidents, not to mention disappointments and heartbreaks. Cancer was one of many difficult experiences that we had survived, yet it caught us unprepared.

First, there are the impossible questions that cancer raises. Most patients ask: "Why me?" "Will I die?" There are no adequate answers, but those questions won't go away. With the prospect of survival, we face different and equally imponderable questions, questions so profound that we are embarrassed to ask them: What is the meaning of life . . . and death? . . . my life, my death? What do I want it to be? And, Even if I knew what "it" was, could I make it happen?

At the core of our experience is a revelation: although there may be a cure for our cancer, there are no simple answers to life's great questions. And surviving cancer throws those questions right in our faces. They are the questions that have occupied great minds throughout all recorded time. No wonder we have trouble with them.

However, the questions are only part of the problem for cancer survivors. Surviving other traumas prompts soul-searching, but it occurs after the threat has passed. As trauma survivors, we may be wounded, but we know that we'll live. As cancer survivors, we hope we are cured and we proceed *as if* we are, but we cannot be sure. Our outcomes are unknown for so long that we are forced to search our souls *while* we are painfully uncertain of our fate. That is why limbo is a cruel pun: it is a place and a dance, and both are difficult.

Discovering Limbo

The two of us assumed that "limbo" was part of Glenna's private language, until we reflected on the survivor interviews. Other survivors not only had their own language for the painful uncertainty of life after cancer, they described a remarkably consistent sequence of emotional states. These states roughly correspond to the phases of treatment and recovery. There is a momentary blinding fear with diagnosis, followed by a period of optimism and determination that carries people through treatment. When treatment is complete, people are surprised and disappointed that their clarity and confidence do not transfer into daily life. Recognizing these emotional landmarks helped us orient ourselves. Both the unexpected "high" of treatment and the unexpected "low" of daily life had contributed to our confusion. Limbo was beginning to make sense. We felt less alone because other survivors had been there, too.

We had all believed that if we could just survive, everything would be all right. We had expected to pick up our lives and go on, as if nothing had really changed, but that didn't work. Like it or not, our lives had changed. Forever. After cancer, we were suspended, not between heaven and hell but between life and death. Before cancer, our lives were based on an admittedly absurd and absolutely human assumption: we were immortal. During treatment, we operated on the equally absurd belief that our will to live could determine our fate. After cancer, all bets were off.

With cancer, we lost our certainty, and that loss was deeply disturbing. Ironically, it was not until we resumed our daily lives that we registered the loss. We were experiencing a form of grief that we now suspect is common among cancer survivors, but we did not recognize the symptoms, and we did not yet appreciate their source. Everyone who survives cancer enters a private terra incognita. This unknown land is paradoxically what was once home ground.

Dancing in Limbo

Just as a metaphor of place helped us get our emotional bearings, a metaphor of dance guided us through this strange new reality. Surviving cancer is like learning a new dance. The dance looks much easier than it is. Sometimes the lessons are more work than fun—especially in the beginning. Furthermore, like the limbo, the dance of life after cancer requires both strength and flexibility. It is also foreign. At first, the movements and the rhythms are unfamiliar, cancer survivors feel awkward and out of sync with the music. With enough time and practice, and a few tips from more experienced dancers, they begin to get the swing of it. Ultimately, the dance flows, as if it came naturally. Even more important, it can be fun. But don't be fooled. Dancing is an art, and no art comes easily.

The dance is our lives after cancer. This book lays out its basic steps. Although each of us creates his or her own dance, it is useful to know the fundamental elements, and it is reassuring to know that all survivors struggle to master them.

The Dance:
Chapter by Chapter, Step by Step

This chapter has been your introduction to limbo. Chapter Two explores why we survivors feel confused and disoriented when treatment ends, and we wake up in limbo. It explains the psychological defenses that protect us from our fear and help-lessness. As we become knowledgeable about our defenses, we can both appreciate their usefulness and allow more of our inner experience into our consciousness. Chapter Three looks at the first question most cancer patients ask: Why me? It examines why we can't stop wondering about the meaning of our illness and, ultimately, the meaning of our lives. To understand and accept what has happened is the first element of the dance. Chapter Four confronts survivor anxiety, looking at fears of recurrence and the wisdom in our worries. With insight and practice, we begin to live with uncertainty. Chapter Five looks at the visible and invisible losses that each survivor must grieve in order to get on with life. This is the step that cannot be skipped if we are to begin to dance. Chapter Six reminds us that living with fear and grief requires courage. We will be tempted to sidestep the dance and fall back on illusions of control. If we master this temptation, we will be able to balance the uncer-tainty of life and the limits of our control without falling into despair. Chapter Seven examines the effect of survivor issues on our most important relationships. Most cancer survivors appre-ciate their families and close friends more deeply than ever before. At this point in the dance, we are ready to fully reen-gage with the significant people in our lives, to join in social dancing. Finally, Chapter Eight looks at how we are changed by the certain knowledge that we are mortal. We don't have time or energy to waste. As we reinvest our energy in life after cancer, we answer the ultimate questions of existence with sim-plicity and courage. We make sense of life. Thus we re-create lives of purpose and meaning. We dance in limbo.

As you read these chapters, you will hear two distinct voices: Glenna's in Chapters Two, Three, Five, and Eight; Lisa's in Chapters Four, Six, Seven, and the Resources. Both of us worked on Chapter One. Our writing reflects our differences in personality and style as well as our contrasting perspectives. Glenna is a long-term survivor, while Lisa's survival is recent. We hope that our differences strengthen the book, just as they enrich our friendship.

Since we cannot be with you during the lonely and confusing moments that are an inescapable part of life after cancer, we hope that you will find our experiences and those of other cancer survivors reassuring: despite what you may be feeling, you are not crazy, and you are certainly not alone.

2

Waking Up in Limbo

I kept a diary during my time with cancer. The entries are filled with raw terror and blind hope, but the emphasis is on hope. Life was wonderful. If I could just survive, everything would be fine. I would never waste my time and energy on everyday hassles. I now knew what was important and what was not. I had attained wisdom—the hard way.

A year later, I was alive and healthy. I sat in our new home trying to write as workers remodeled the place. The phone rang. An old friend asked how I was doing and out poured my petty complaints: construction workers everywhere, noise and dust, chaos all around me. I longed for the comfort and order of the old house. What was wrong with me? "I promised myself that if I survived cancer I would never let this stuff get me down. Now I'm a basket case over nothing," I lamented. "No," my friend counseled. "You're just still human." But I didn't feel human. In fact, I identified with my dog, Miguel. The workers had demolished the master bedroom, which Miguel considered his domain. In his agitation, Miguel would pace back and forth between my office and the barrier of heavy plastic at the other end of the hallway, where the bedroom door had been. There he would sit for hours, banished from his world. Confused and whining, he would come back to me, his eyes pleading, "Let me into my familiar place." He had done nothing to deserve this, but I could neither explain it to him, nor set it right.

GLENNA

13

Poor Miguel. He was in limbo—and so was I. Miguel was dislocated in physical space; I was lost within myself. Neither of us could understand what had happened, and the harder we tried to return to what had been, the more distressed we felt. The need for home and comfort, for one's own familiar place, is elemental. Miguel wanted his old room back, and so did I, but more than that, I wanted my old life back.

During the crisis of diagnosis and treatment, I had not appeared frightened or depressed. I was optimistic, determined, compulsively well organized, and in control. After treatment, I let my guard down. I was not only human and therefore vulnerable to the normal irritants of life, I was raw from my recent scrape with death. I was extra sensitive to feelings of disorientation and loss.

Living in a construction site was too much like surviving cancer. I mourned the loss of my old house with added force because I did not know that I was mourning the loss of my old familiar sense of self. Despite my optimism, I knew, for the first time, that I was mortal. I was not at home in a world that included my own inevitable death. No wonder I felt lost in a new house that was being remodeled. My sense of self was undergoing major renovation.

My friend's compassion cut me to the quick: still alive and therefore still human. Ouch! During the crisis, I had felt superhuman. Why couldn't that feeling last? The Pollyanna quality of my journal entries is a clue. My heightened sense of well-being in the face of death was based in denial—of death and of the complexities of life. My defenses had served me well, but it was time to give them up.

What Is Limbo?

As the first chapter began to explain, limbo is the rest of our lives as cancer survivors. Ultimately, our task is to live fully and actively in the face of uncertainty and mortality. However, when we wake up in limbo, we do not yet know this; we do not know what is going on. We certainly do not question where we are:

we can see that we are at home, at work, or with family and friends. Why don't we feel the comfort of old familiar ways? All we know is that something is not right; this is not what we expected. We are in limbo, but we don't know that yet.

We enter limbo when we are diagnosed, but in our shock and terror, we don't notice. There are too many other things on our minds. Diagnosis and treatment are so overwhelming, they demand our full attention. During treatment, there is an elegant economy to our thoughts. There is no reason to worry about the future. We may not have one.

When treatment is complete and successful, then all we can do is wait. *Now* we can afford to worry. We want to count ourselves among the lucky, but we can't be sure. The nagging uncertainty puts a damper on our joy. We try to pick up our lives and go on, as if nothing has really changed, but that doesn't work either.

There is no easy awakening in limbo. I knew I was in pain, but I tried to carry on. In my family, the rules were rigid: good and gracious manners were required at all times. Although I had never completely lived up to this code of honor, in my late thirties I was still bound by it. Waking up in limbo meant breaking all the rules. So it took me a long time to admit what was going on.

Lisa's family had different customs. She woke up wailing her distress. Either way, we were both disoriented and distraught. My feelings were disguised while Lisa's were exposed, but we each thought something was wrong with us. Given the benefit of hindsight and the experiences of other cancer survivors, we now understand what was wrong. We were in limbo, and we could no longer avoid the pain.

Nancy's experience was a classic journey to limbo. Nancy developed breast cancer when she was in her mid fifties. She discovered the lump while she was on vacation with her husband. She kept the finding to herself, hoping it was nothing, but went to see her doctor as soon as they got home. When a lumpectomy revealed more widespread disease, she had a mastectomy followed by chemotherapy. "I experienced a high during chemotherapy," she said. "I felt strong and challenged—a great sense of euphoria, even though the chemicals were poisoning my body as well as the cancer. After the treatments, when I returned to my 'other life,' I felt very vulnerable and depressed. I was no longer actively engaged in 'cancer combat,' and a dreadful fear engulfed me: when would the other shoe drop?"

Like Nancy, Lisa and I were feeling bad right on time, but neither of us knew the schedule. We had expected to feel bad during treatment and good when it was over, but that's not how limbo works. Limbo is governed by an emotional logic that defies survivors' rational expectations.

The Logic of Limbo

Once you wake up to it, you find that limbo has its own logic, its own "normal" sequence of feelings.

The Unexpected High

With the diagnosis of cancer, most patients feel terror. However, for many of us who have survived, that blind fear bordering on panic is quickly replaced with hope. Fear may break through at moments, but our dominant sense remains that of hope. We are confident that we can do whatever it takes to survive. We often possess a clarity and an odd calm, while those who love us are worried and agitated. Despite the rigors of treatment, many cancer patients experience this "high." Our defenses are working overtime, and they are doing a beautiful job.

The blind hope and single-minded purpose that carry us through the treatment phase also fool us and others. We seem to be in control, and what proves worse, we may actually believe that we are in control of our fate. The high of treatment is based on sheer determination and strong defenses, an intoxicating combination that cannot last.

Lost in Limbo

During treatment, our focus is narrow and clear: obliterate the cancer. When the job is done, we lose our focus. Suddenly, cancer no longer defines us—structuring our time, consuming our energy—and we are at loose ends. At the same time, all the people who have cared for us go on about their business, leaving us to ours. We are alone.

As we resume our daily lives, we feel disoriented. Something is amiss, but we don't know what it is. Most of us have no energy; some of us are irritable and depressed. Fears of a recurrence start creeping into our thoughts. Simultaneously, real life with all its mundane urgency demands our attention. We are overwhelmed by the smallest things.

I have always been a morning person. I love the sky at dawn, and my mind has always been alert and active at that time. But for months, I did not want to wake up. Whatever the day might bring, I did not feel up to it. I remember wanting to rip the phone from the wall. Every time it rang, I felt assaulted. Someone was wanting something more from me, and I had nothing left to give.

In addition to our disorientation and depression, we begin to experience more anxiety. Our moods may vacillate between confusion and fear. Fears of recurrence begin to dominate our thoughts, and we may sometimes feel obsessed with death. These are the fears that we have held in check. Now that we are stronger, they can emerge.

Just when we expected to feel relieved, we don't. The irony is painful: we thought this would be the easy part! We may assume our feelings are the aftermath of treatment, and in a way we're right, but they have a deeper source. The reversal of expected feeling states is the hallmark of survivor grief, as yet unrecognized by us. For the moment, we are lost in limbo. And we're lost, in large measure, because our defenses are still in force, keeping us removed from our inner life of thoughts and feelings

The Disappointing Low

Too much is happening, and since we were not expecting any of it, we are not prepared. We didn't expect to lose our sense of purpose when treatment ended. Not when it had all seemed so clear. How could daily life throw us, after all that we've been through? We feel estranged from others because they do not understand, yet we do not understand ourselves well enough to explain our condition to them. Furthermore, we may not want the people we love the most to know just how bad we feel. Still more surprising, and at the bottom of it all, there is grief. We have begun to feel its nagging pain. It is the low point of limbo.

Survivor grief is a paradox. It seems wrong to grieve when we have got what we most wanted—another chance at life. Furthermore, the early high deceived us. Normal grief does not begin on a high. So the process is in motion before we recognize it. Furthermore, we are grieving major losses. Most obviously, we mourn lost body parts or functions. But survivors also grieve a deeper loss. Our most comforting illusions are gone. We are both mortal and vulnerable, and we know it beyond a doubt. It is simply awful.

Working Through

At this low point, we can't do anything about losing our focus and sense of purpose. We just have to tolerate feeling lost for a while. The big questions will not go away, but we also cannot answer them yet. Ultimately, a new sense of purpose will flow from our answers, but we are not there yet. Much of the real world will not go away either, although many survivors begin to make changes in their daily lives—cutting back on work or on social obligations. Our grief has a life of its own. We need to recognize it, respect it, and allow it to run its natural course.

This is, of course, more easily said than done. I had difficulty with these first, intense phases of limbo—both because of the rules in my head and because the timing of life's events can be perverse. The first nine months after treatment were a seemingly endless string of hardships, including my father-in-law's unexpected death. That period culminated in an auto accident in which my youngest stepson was nearly killed. The phone rang in the middle of the night: "This is the admissions nurse at Presbyterian Emergency Room. Your son has been in an accident. We need you to come down." I drove to the hospital in a trance and waited through the night as doctors sewed Kyle's face together and set his broken arm and leg.

Kyle had been thrown from the car, but he would live. Alone in the dark of an OR waiting room, I realized that something had happened that I could never fix. I went numb with grief. And I did what I have always done: put one foot in front of the other and move on. Weeks later, as I drove Kyle to one of his many doctor's appointments, I ran a stoplight. There were no other cars in sight, but Kyle screamed in fear. I pulled to the side of the road and put my head on the steering wheel. I hadn't even seen the light. I felt as if I were failing at everything, including mothering. I had a badly injured son who needed me, and my own feelings were getting in the way.

That was more than a decade ago. Kyle is nearly thirty now and a talented documentary filmmaker. I sent him an early draft of this book because I trust his artistic judgment. He wrote back: "It was sad for me to read this because . . . I have never been aware of all that you went through. I feel a little ashamed. As if, at the time, I was too self-absorbed to register it all."

Kyle was a normal adolescent when I had cancer, busy with the work of growing up. He still believed that he was invulnerable and therefore so was I. By the time he had the accident, I was grieving my own brush with death, my father-in-law's death, and then his near death. I was in an overload of grief. During the intervening years, we have each worried that we did not do enough. As we talk about it now, we realize that we each did our best, and it was good enough.

We're Not Alone in Limbo

Although I hope that my overload of grief is atypical, the repeated traumas hammered away at my defenses and, ultimately, forced me to look at the hard truths of survival. The difficulty of waking up in limbo seems obvious once it is stated, but it is seldom clear when we are in it. Our thoughts are muddled; our feelings are raw. We have vague sensations and fleeting images but few words for waking up in limbo. The cancer survivors Lisa and I interviewed had their own images for the nagging uncertainty of limbo. One characterized her life after cancer as "a wait-and-see game." Several thought of themselves as "a time bomb waiting to go off" or as "living on borrowed time." Another worried, "I don't know if I'm on death row or not." While these metaphors seemed to focus on whether or not one was cured, other metaphors indicated a more generalized alteration in view. One person commented that "life is a crapshoot." The free-floating quality of death anxiety is captured in another woman's observation that she felt "untethered."

Some of us feel a hint of limbo near the end of treatment, as we are literally untethered. The oxygen tube is taken away, the last intravenous tube removed, and we feel anxious instead of relieved. I remember my paradoxical reaction when my tracheostomy tube was removed. I hated that thing. It was the worst part of treatment, and I counted the days until it could come out. But after it was pulled, I went into a funk—the only low I experienced during treatment. For about twenty-four hours, I felt bereft, but I didn't make the connection between the removal of the tube and my feelings. However, another survivor made the connection. With a double mastectomy and chemotherapy three years behind her, Charlotte continues to take tamoxifen daily: "To me, it's like a lifeline, and I'm clinging to it. . . . Taking my medicine is like a security blanket. I feel sorry for people who don't have something like that."

Barbara, a breast cancer survivor in her early forties, described what it was like to lose the sense of security that her doctors had provided her. "After my second surgery, my surgeon said, 'You don't need to see me any more.' This was a man I'd seen every six months for three years. Then my radiologist said, 'You don't need to see me any more, either.' I felt like they had been watching out for me, and suddenly I thought, 'Oh, my god! I'm on my own. How am I going to know if I'm okay?' It was a very scary feeling."

When we wake up in limbo, the sense of disconnection is profound, as if fundamental ties have come undone. When we wake up, we are alone, acutely aware of our vulnerability and helplessness and filled with the dread of recurrence. No wonder we wake in fits and starts; the whole would overwhelm us.

However, with a little distance and the genuine reassurance of a hopeful prognosis, we need our defenses less. In addition, most of us simply cannot remain on guard at all times. Reality begins to slip in. We are waking up to the painful thoughts and feelings that our defenses had covered up. We are finally seeing limbo.

As we wake up, we have little insight into the defenses that have brought us this far and less understanding of the grief that is ahead. In the next section of this chapter, I will examine the defenses that protect us during treatment, so we can both appreciate how we got to limbo and understand ourselves better for the future. As we increase our tolerance for the bad feelings that are part of the reality of surviving cancer, we need our defenses *less*, but we will always need them.

How We Got Here: Psychological Defenses

We all need emotional protection, and that is what our defenses offer. Like an umbrella on a rainy day or an overcoat on a cold one, our defenses keep us dry and warm through psychological bad weather. Unlike an umbrella or coat, they are invisible (especially to the user) and automatic—no levers, no buttons. Defenses are just there when we need them, and we are unaware of them even as we use them. For this reason, psychologists describe them as unconscious, and for this reason, they are difficult to talk about. We are attempting to explain something that, by definition, we are oblivious to.

Defenses protect us from the outside world and from ourselves. When the world hits us too hard, our defenses deflect the blow. When our own thoughts and feelings would be totally unacceptable if we knew about them, our defenses enable us not to know. We are unaware of both the defense mechanism and whatever it protects us from.

It is fashionable to put down defenses. We are more likely to say, "Now don't get defensive," than to appreciate their smooth operation. In fact, we all have defenses, and we all need them. In competitive sports, defensive strategies and skills are valued. Our psychological strategies and skills deserve similar respect.

Surviving cancer taught me to appreciate my defenses. For perhaps the first time in my life, I realized how skillfully my mind protected me from emotional overload. My terror of dying from cancer was mysteriously self-limiting. I would be engulfed by fear, literally shaking and crying, and then I would just space out or my thoughts would turn to something pleasant. I didn't will these shifts. They just happened. I would stop crying and go on with whatever needed to be done. I simply followed along, trusting the wisdom within me. Such "inner wisdom" is simply another term for defenses in action.

Although we are seldom aware of our own defenses, their workings may become clear after the fact, when we reflect upon them or when they break down. In *Girl, Interrupted*, novelist Susanna Kaysen describes the emotional breakdown and psychiatric hospitalization that "interrupted" her transition from adolescence to adulthood. "Something had been peeled back, a covering or shell that works to protect us. I couldn't decide whether the covering was something on me or something attached to every thing in the world. It didn't matter, really; wherever it had been, it wasn't there anymore." Without our defenses, we cannot function in the world.

At best, our defenses work smoothly, but they are not effortless. And that is the key point of this discussion: we feel bad, and we do not know why. The simple fact is that we feel a little bad when our defenses work well, we feel awful when they don't. Effective defenses use a lot of psychic energy. The more heavily we need to defend ourselves, the more energy is required. It is exhausting. But that is not the worst. Since our defenses are human, they are never perfect. A little bit of what we cannot tolerate knowing always leaks through, and sometimes a lot gets through. At those times, we are flooded. Psychologically, we are drowning, and we feel it.

For Lisa and me, the best offense has been a strong defense. Seriously. Understanding our defensive strategies and skills, and then respecting them, has helped us cope more effectively with much of life, including the inevitable fears of recurrence that plague all cancer survivors.

Based on our own experience and that of the survivors we interviewed, we have identified four common and useful defenses among cancer survivors: denial, dissociation, displacement, and repression. Each technique has both benefits and costs, and they are best illustrated by examples of real defenses used by real cancer survivors. When it comes to defenses, we all know more than we know that we know.

Nothing Happened: Denial

Have you ever had a friend or colleague talk to you about a shared experience, only to realize that you don't remember it? "No," you think, "that didn't happen." But the friend persists with the story, recalling so much plausible detail that you begin to wonder, "What is going on here? Was I out of the room at a crucial moment? Did my attention wander?" Perhaps, but if the event is emotionally loaded for you, the answer to what is going on is probably denial. When we are in denial, we simply do not see what we are not prepared to see, nor hear what we are not ready to hear. By this method, we guard against intolerable realities.

Other people's denial is always more apparent than our own. It would not be denial if we saw what we were doing. I mentioned the sore in my mouth to my husband several times, and reacting as if I were his mother, the hypochondriac, he ignored me. After my dentist had seen the lesion and arranged for my biopsy that same afternoon, I drove to my husband's office to deliver the bad news. When I arrived, Curtis already knew. Our dentist, in his concern, had called immediately. As Curtis tells the story, the conversation went like this: "Curtis, this is Jim Williams. I've just examined Glenna, and I think she has an oral cancer. I'm sending her directly to an oral surgeon for a biopsy." To which Curtis replied, "You must have the wrong number. I don't have a client by that name." Our dentist said, "No, Curtis, I'm talking about your wife, Glenna." Curtis said, "I'm sure you have the wrong number." This same exchange was repeated several more times before my husband was able to hear what our dentist was trying to tell him.

Unfortunately, of all the defenses, denial gets the least respect. Denial is our first defense, the root from which all the others grow. Although we may develop more mature defenses, denial is the one we all fall back on when things get bad enough. For some people, denial is always the primary defense. Either way, denial is always with us.

Nothing makes the value of denial clearer than its loss. As we were preparing this chapter, Lisa confessed, "Every so often, I'm chilled by my knowledge that I may not survive this melanoma." The rest of the time, denial protects her from the chill. The beauty of defenses became even clearer when Lisa could not remember having said this! (That useful forgetting is repression, and I will talk about it soon.)

The cold fact is that both Lisa and I will die. So will you. If not from cancer, then from something else, some other day. There is no way around it: every life ends in death. As obvious as this seems, we all deny the inevitability of our own deaths almost all of the time. Intellectually we know it, but emotionally we don't really get it, except in jolts and jokes. George Burns has made a late-life career of one-liners about death: he hates growing old, but it beats the alternative; he doesn't think he'll die . . . it's already been done.

A friend loves to tell of her spunky grandmother who, in her nineties, began to admit the possibility of death. "If I die," she said, but never "when I die." As we laugh at other people's denial, we also laugh with them. How thoroughly human to deny our own death.

Secondary Denial

We talk about denial as if it were an all-or-nothing phenomenon when it may not be. Many cancer survivors are masters of partial (or secondary) denial. We may have recognized a symptom of our cancer and gone to a doctor promptly without ever admitting that it could be cancer. We may have accepted the diagnosis but not the possibility that we could die. We may have known the odds but believed that we would beat them. We may now recognize that we had a life-threatening illness but deny that it could recur. These are all examples of secondary denial: we admit the fact while obliterating the intolerable implications of that fact. We take in only as much reality as we can tolerate.

Denial is most useful in this form. When it is partial, not complete, and when it is the initial phase of an adjustment, not a permanent state, denial is invaluable. Several of the survivors interviewed described their use of denial at the time of diagnosis. Ann, a fitness instructor in her early sixties, said, "My initial reaction was 'I can't believe it!' And my other reaction was that since it was a fluke that my cancer was found, I felt very lucky." As she openly rejected the diagnosis of a melanoma, she simultaneously redefined the horrible news as good luck. After she saw herself as a lucky person, she could then accept the diagnosis—presumably a lucky person would survive the cancer.

Benefits of Denial

Denial buys us time to adjust to a hard reality without our having to *do* anything—since there is *nothing* to do anything about. We can then absorb the bad news in small doses, a fleeting thought, a partial recognition. Slowly, we work up to a fuller dose of reality, while avoiding an overdose. I used denial in just this way. Although I suspected that the sore in my mouth was cancer before it was diagnosed, I used secondary denial throughout treatment. I believed that despite the fact that I had a frequently lethal form of cancer, I would survive. Before my demoralizing trip to the medical school library, I primed myself. If I could find just one article with one survivor, I would be that lone survivor. My secondary denial had many breaks in it, including my time in the library and the several times that I curled up with Curtis on the sofa and simply cried out all my fears—of dying, of leaving him, of never seeing the children grown and on their own. My denial was incomplete, but it was there when I needed it the most.

Ann used denial in her own creative and useful way. She noticed the mole on her upper thigh, but did nothing about it. When she saw her dermatologist for another problem, she casually mentioned the mole. He removed it immediately, and one week later she "could not believe" that it had been a melanoma. Her initial denial was partial, or she would not have asked the doctor to check the mole, and she continued in that mode. She had regular check-ups for five years despite her belief that "the chapter was closed." By denying the possibility of further problems, she saved herself five years of anxiety. In that fifth year, a metastasis to her lymph system was detected, and she had more extensive surgery. Now Ann talks frankly about the fear of death that settles upon her when she crawls into bed at night. Yet most of the time, she tolerates the fear, maintaining a satisfying marriage, an active career, loving relationships with her children, and many friendships. Denial works.

Then Why Do We Feel Bad?

If denial works so well, why do we feel so bad? In order to understand our dilemma, let's take a closer look at denial. As survivors, we have faced death, and once faced, it can no longer be completely denied. It is as if the denial of death were a magic spell. Once the spell is broken, it cannot be cast again. Any reminder of death, and there are many in everyday life, makes us realize what we have lost.

Just as I thought my life was getting back to normal, my father-in-law died unexpectedly. When I came home from my first business trip following my cancer surgery, Curtis met me at the airport, and as we walked to the car, he said, "My father died today." All I wanted to do was scream, "NO!" It was late at night. We stood in a covered parking lot. I wanted my voice to fill the entire space, blocking out everything but my denial. Instead, I sat in silence as we drove to my husband's childhood home for the wake the following morning. I can still see the hearse coming slowly down the long driveway. Four men slide a sleek steel coffin out and across the yard. I hold the door open. Somehow it's the burnished metal that undoes me. My father-in-law had stood at my bedside, confident of his own health, afraid that I would die. Instead, he is dead. How can this be? My chest aches with the certain knowledge that it is— that the body in that coffin could be me.

After we wake up in limbo, we face the rest of our lives stripped of the protective barrier between ourselves and death. Death is real and close at hand. Although we may want to proceed as if nothing has changed, for most of us such efforts are only partially successful. We cannot escape the fact that we know how vulnerable we are and that others know that truth as well. Most of us cannot get life insurance, and the rejection slips are nasty reminders that the whole world knows that we are mortal. Even when denial is our preferred mode of adaptation, the real world does not play along.

A further reason that we feel bad is embedded in the irony of denial. Although denial means not knowing, effective denial requires that we know exactly what to deny. It takes skill and hard work not to see, hear, feel, or think important things that are happening in and around us. Such directed use of psychic energy has its costs. At best, it is tiring. We have less energy for everything else, and we have no idea why we are so tired. At worst, denial leaves us so out of touch with reality that meaningful activities and relationships become impossible. This is exactly what happens with the alcoholic who is in denial of his or her disease. When we cannot see, hear, or speak the truth, we are severely handicapped.

The trick in using denial is to get the benefits at a reasonable cost. For most of us, this happens automatically. Both Lisa and I have learned to trust and value our own defensive ways.

However, there is also an important role for survivors' friends, family, and caregivers. First and foremost, these important people in our lives need to be aware of their own tendency to deny the reality that something awful could happen to us. If they are able to manage their own denial, they can often help us with ours—very gently. They can keep track of the schedule for follow-up appointments—since we just might forget about them. They can be alert to signs and symptoms of a recurrence. They can also monitor our anxiety levels and encourage us to check out anything that is worrying us, or them.

All of us need to accept denial as a given and respect its usefulness and its power. Do not try to break through someone else's denial. It simply won't work, and you risk driving the person away. My own friends are on to me: when one of them thinks that I'm ignoring something I should be attending to, she or he says, "Just do it for me. You don't want me worrying unnecessarily, do you?" Oh, they're clever. They know that the caretaker in me will see to their feelings, even when my denial would prevent me from taking care of my own health.

Fortunately, most of us are a lot like Ann. Our denial kicks in when we really need it, and our realism kicks in as soon as we can handle it. In order to function, we move in and out of deeply felt awareness of our own mortality. This movement is accomplished through the intermittent use of denial and also of other defensive strategies.

This Cannot Be Happening to Me: Dissociation

Dissociation may be the most common reaction to the diagnosis of cancer. Many of the survivors Lisa and I interviewed spontaneously described periods of dissociation during diagnosis and treatment. In describing her initial shock, Ellen, an educational consultant and another survivor of melanoma, said, "I just felt absolutely detached from myself." That sense of detachment is the hallmark of dissociation. Unlike denial and repression, dissociation is a technique we often notice in ourselves even though observers may be unaware of our absence from what is happening around us. Stan, an attorney who had a mastectomy for breast cancer in his late fifties, recalled that when his doctor said, "I'm sorry. It's malignant," he immediately dissociated. "I didn't even think the doctor was talking to me. I didn't relate in any way. I didn't have the feeling that this was me he was talking to." For the moment, we simply are not ourselves.

Although we hear the information accurately and may even remember it, when we dissociate, we aren't really there. Emotionally, we flee the scene. Barbara's language captures the essence of dissociation when she speaks of herself but uses a generic "you" rather than "I" or "me": "At that point, your mind just goes on hold. You don't know what to think. You don't know what to do. You just sort of become numb." In our numbness and our distance from the self who was diagnosed with cancer, we escape the pain. For a while.

Most of us come back to ourselves, feel the pain, and go on. Ellen remembered the time-lapse, "[At first], I was watching my life, and my life was a movie, and I was not in my body. After about a week, it hit me like a ton of bricks. I thought I was going to die." During the period of dissociation, she was insulated from her overwhelming terror of death. When she reentered her body and her life, she was able to function despite the heavy weight of fear. She called a physician friend, gathered information, and sought appropriate treatment.

Similarly, at the time of a possible metastasis of her breast cancer to her ovaries, Dorothy noted: "I'd be having this very logical conversation with the doctor, and we'd be talking about me, my life. Maybe my life is going to be over pretty soon. Wait a minute. Rewind this video. I don't like it." Again, there is the sense of watching, not being, ourselves—and of watching ourselves watching. As Dorothy described it: "Every once in a while, it is this mind shift to think that you're actually talking about yourself. It feels very weird." Fortunately, Dorothy, a business consultant in her forties, had a scare, not a recurrence.

Dissociation is both weird and common. Most of the survivors were aware of dissociating at the time of diagnosis or of a possible recurrence, but intermittent sensations of distance from the self who had cancer may become an enduring part of our adjustment to the terrifying fact. After more than ten years, I still experience the time warp of dissociation. Much of the time, I feel completely connected to my past. Sometimes I feel that it was yesterday. At other times, it seems so far away that I almost believe it didn't happen to me. When the survivors were asked what had most surprised them in their experience with cancer, the majority said, "That it happened to *me*." Dissociation lingers.

Some cancer survivors train themselves to dissociate in order to manage their ongoing anxiety. Through meditation or other forms of guided imagery, we may learn to create an inner state of peace, an imaginary safe place to which we can retreat when our feelings threaten to overwhelm us. Books and movies can distract us and alter our mood. Or we may simply "space out" when we need to. All of these forms of dissociation allow us to escape our pain. Getting some distance when we need it is helpful.

However, some researchers, including Christine Dunkel-Schetter and her colleagues, emphasize that if escapism becomes a habit or if we augment our natural abilities with drugs or alcohol, we harm ourselves. There is a growing body of evidence that dissociation is a natural reaction in crisis and adaptive as such. However, research on the victims of the Oakland/Berkeley firestorm found that dissociation impedes the grief process that is essential to a lasting recovery from trauma. Brief periods of dissociation, especially in the midst of crisis, give us some relief, something like a valve on a pressure cooker, and may allow us to function better than we otherwise could. But prolonged dissociative states and deliberate dissociation, especially through the use of alcohol or drugs, actually hinder our recovery.

I Have So Many
Other Worries: Displacement

As we live with the ebb and flow of death anxiety, we may find ourselves worrying more than we used to—about our jobs, our houses, our cars, our kids' grades, anything *except* our cancer. We manage overwhelming anxiety about our own deaths by transferring the feelings of dread to something else in our lives. The object of our worries is often a metaphor for loss or death. My horrible feelings about moving into a new house were clearly displaced from my experience with cancer. A year later, I could resent the hell out of the workers who remodeled my house while still feeling grateful to the doctors and nurses who had done so many invasive things to my body.

Jeannette was having shortness of breath at the time of her interview. Since this retired professor in her late seventies had survived lung cancer four years earlier, this was a minor symptom with major implications. After revealing her concern, she quickly stated, "I'm not going to think about it," and seemingly changed the subject. She said, "I'm worried about when the hell am I going to sell this house and move into a place that's more accessible to public transportation." She spoke with concern about the problems of maintaining her house, not her health.

Such decoy worries allow us to experience some of our feelings without being overwhelmed by the real thing. Jeannette believed that "it would be masochistic" to worry about her health, but acknowledged, "I tend to get much more involved with practical problems about which I can do something. I may agonize about those decisions." These less vital concerns carry the agonizing burden of her powerlessness in the face of lung cancer.

We can all be reasonably confident that life after cancer will present enough problems to occupy us—apart from our cancer. There will be a ready supply of issues onto which we can displace our death anxiety. All the problems that plagued me in the first year after cancer were real and serious. However, I can now see that my reactions to them were colored by my awful dread of a recurrence and by the grief I could hardly bear.

Sounding much like me, Charlotte, a housewife and school board member, noted, "I really don't have time to worry about the cancer because we have so many other things going on in the family. I don't think we create these other worries per se, but they do prevent us from thinking about the cancer." Then she reflected more deeply: "We have an expression in Swedish that says you tippy-toe around something, like a hot bowl of cereal, because you don't want to touch it. And I wonder if we don't want to touch the cancer issue."

When we asked Norm, a roofing contractor in his forties, if he was aware of worrying more about things other than his cancer during the first several years after his melanoma was diagnosed, his answer was priceless: "You mean like displacing the fear or something? No more than usual. I'm a worrier. I come from a long line of worriers. We're champions in my family, so I worry about anything." He later provided an elegant example of displaced death anxiety. When one of the women in his melanoma support group died, Norm went to the memorial service with other group members. It was raining as they drove to the cemetery, and Norm confessed that he felt indifferent about Nancy and her death, despite the strong bond of caring he had always felt for her. With the first fall rain, all he could think about were the roofs he had repaired the past summer. Would they leak? He worried about water leaking into his customers' homes, not about his cancer spreading as Nancy's had, and certainly not about his fears of death leaking into consciousness. Nancy got a leak, and now she was dead.

It is worth noting that few of the survivors interviewed were aware of displacing their anxiety. The process works because it remains unconscious. However, the survivors who openly worried about a recurrence and lamented their feelings of uncertainty about life in general, appeared to worry less about other issues. More worries about work and relationships and houses and who knows what were expressed by the survivors who disavowed death anxiety.

When Lisa and I find ourselves worrying excessively over minor things or worrying habitually about the same thing, we have learned to consider the possibility that we are displacing deeper concerns about our cancer. Then we ask, "Why is this worrying me *now*? What could this be saying about me and cancer?" We ask what else is going on at this time. Monthly checkup? Annual physical? Anniversary of diagnosis or treatment? Bad news about the health of a friend or family member? These are all events that activate death anxiety. We cannot eliminate this anxiety, but labeling it helps, and we can often stop worrying about all the things that are *not* the problem.

Just Don't Think About It (and It Won't Go Away): Repression

When we do not deny horrible realities, we can still repress them. Lisa confessed her chilling fear of dying and promptly forgot that she had ever made the confession. That forgetting is repression. When repression is at work, we really cannot remember what's bothering us. We lose the connection between real events and our feelings about them. The event gets lost. The feelings stay behind, nagging at us. Many of the cancer survivors described their use of repression. Several of them were aware that their minds were playing tricks on them; others were not.

Early in her interview, Judy, a tour consultant in her early fifties, made it clear that working her way through the medical system to get her breast cancer diagnosed and treated had been frustrating despite her total satisfaction with both of her surgeons. As she tried to reconstruct the series of events that led to her diagnosis, she chuckled, "Funny how this all blurs in my memory." Then she interrupted her own train of thought, "That's not how it happened. Oh, how you block this stuff out." She went on to tell a horror story about the incompetent and insensitive treatment she received from the doctor who reviewed her mammogram, concluding, "God, I'd forgotten about that."

Along with a curious forgetfulness, repression is character-ized by a relentless emphasis on the positive. My upbeat jour-nal entries smack of repression. The perfect motto for this defense is the refrain, "Accentuate the positive, eliminate the negative." Several survivors seemed to live by this rule. It wasn't a conscious choice; it was simply their way of experiencing life. Stan described his breast cancer and mastectomy as "an ex-tremely useful thing that has happened in my life. I don't think of it as a negative, I think of it more as a positive."

Stan was determined to eliminate the negative. He talked about the New Age books he had read which had "all been very healing and very uplifting." They helped him "not feel despair." Stan then said, "I had one, maybe two nights in which I couldn't sleep because I was afraid that I was about to die. That was right after the diagnosis. I had one night when I was really a basket case . . . uh, I had about three." He clearly intended to accentuate the positive, but his disavowal of despair brought back the memory of a dreadful night, and as he thought out loud, one bad night led to memories of several more. In the midst of this painful reverie, Stan's mind changed the subject: "This was tougher on my wife. . . . I had much more concern for her than I had for me." Although his con-cern for his wife was genuine, it also provided an escape from his own intolerable feelings. A lot is going on in Stan's active mind, but the negation of his pain, which led by association to memories of just how bad he has felt, is a classic feature of repression.

Most people who think of themselves as strong and who function well in crisis use repression. Socorro was nearly fifty at the time of her interview. She had had breast cancer ten years earlier and remembered no emotional ups or downs after her mastectomy. An instructional aide in her working life, she just wanted information, lots of it, and reassurance from experts whenever she heard bad news about other people with breast cancer. However, four years after her bout with cancer, Socorro had a hemorrhage in her brain. The doctors debated the cause of the bleeding. Was it from a brain tumor—a metastatic spread of her breast cancer? The problem turned out to be a vascular defect, which was successfully repaired, but the episode really scared her and that fright in turn mystified her: "It surprised me . . . because I think of myself as this strong person. Yet I couldn't shake it. I shook the breast cancer and the mastectomy really quickly." She remembered that she had seen a psychotherapist following the brain surgery. The therapist had been "absolutely wonderful," providing the information and reassurance that she had needed. Later in the interview, she reiterated her sense of personal strength, noting that "it was so surprising to me that I would have to go to therapy." She tried to recall how that had happened: "I can't even remember how I found the therapist. I was suicidal. Oh, I forgot that." She wondered out loud, "What was happening? I can't even remember." But then more repressed memories came back, of a sad and disturbing family problem. The whole painful picture came back into focus for her. Briefly. She ended the interview by firmly stating that she would never presume to give another cancer survivor advice because "other people might not be as lucky" as she was. Although Socorro's recognition that her survival holds no guarantee for others is accurate, her formidable ability to forget the unlucky events of her life reveals that the underlying mechanism is repression.

As Socorro's experience illustrates, repression helps us to see ourselves as "strong," but we pay dearly for our strength. In rejecting all "weak" feelings, especially fear and sadness, we reject much that is truly human in ourselves (and others). In essence, if we feel bad, we then feel bad about ourselves for feeling bad.

One of the ways that repression reveals itself is in anniversary reactions. On the same day of the week or at the same time of year as a previous traumatic event, we will feel mysteriously depressed or anxious, although we have given no conscious thought to the trauma. (The most amazing thing is that we often have the anniversary reaction on the exact date!) I first became aware of that phenomenon in the first year after my divorce. I had married my college sweetheart, and five years later, we had divorced. On the exact date of our wedding anniversary, I woke up with the blues. That evening, I told an old friend about my mysterious bad day. My friend pointed out the connection; until then I had not had a clue.

Three of the survivors interviewed described anniversary reactions. Barbara first told us how swiftly her initial diagnosis and treatment had transpired, "I went in on a Thursday for my biopsy, and by the following Thursday, I'd had my surgery." Two and a half years later, when she had decided to have a second and more extensive procedure, she had to wait four weeks for that surgery. Those weeks were hell. "All the fears about surgery and anaesthesia would come to me in the night. I'd be fine, and suddenly I'd become hysterical—usually on Thursday nights. I don't know what it was about Thursday nights, but I'd fall apart." That was an anniversary reaction.

Charlotte is aware that she's vulnerable on the anniversary of her diagnosis and surgery. "I have a little dip right around the anniversary. I don't know if I should be happy that I have lived another year, or sad and apprehensive that I might be one year closer to a recurrence. I have mixed feelings, and I don't know how to react, but it happens every year."

Norm had a profound reaction on his first anniversary, "About a year after the surgery, I just hit bottom. I just wanted to die, you know." Sadly, most of us do know—if not the suicidal depths, the hitting bottom when we least expect it. Just when reason would dictate relief and celebration of a survival milestone, our unreasonable unconscious, with the most accurate clock in town, throws us another curve. Those unexpected curves are the awful essence of waking up in limbo.

Although repression exacts a high price, there is strong social support, even social pressure in its favor. Most of us were encouraged to forget about our illness and get on with life. Undoubtedly, the people who told us "don't dwell on it" and "put it behind you" meant well. However, the underlying message is a destructive one. In part, the speaker is saying, "If you feel bad, I don't want to hear about it." Others may need to protect themselves from our worst fears—and their own. However, instead of saying that, they prescribe repression when our natural aptitude will facilitate more than enough forgetting. The real task in surviving any trauma, including cancer, is, at an appropriate time, to remember and to mourn what we have lost. Only then can we get on with living.

Repression is probably the major reason that cancer survivors are confused by the unexpected bad feelings that surface during the first year after treatment. Without repression, we would expect to feel bad, and we would know why. Something really bad has happened to us. In fact, that is exactly how Judy saw it. When asked if she had felt sad with no apparent reason, she replied, "I felt a lot of sadness during the first year, but there was a very apparent reason." Unlike Judy, many of us "forget" that.

At this painful point in the process, it is important to remind ourselves (and each other) that all of limbo isn't pain. It is the waking up that feels so bad. Nancy said it clearly, "Limbo is forever, but the worst of the awful feeling does pass, in its own time." One of the great truths in psychology and life is Gestalt therapist Fritz Perls's aphorism: "The only way out is through." Damn it, he's right. And the greatest song about limbo is Jimmy Cliff's "Sitting in Limbo." It's time to remember the lines:

> Sittin here in limbo, but I know it won't be long.
> Sittin here in limbo, and I feel like a bird ain't got no
>   song.
> . . . and I'm waitin for the dice to roll . . .
> and I still got a little time to search my soul.
> I can't see where life will lead me,
> but I know where I have been.
> I can't see what life will show me,
> but I know what I have seen.
> . . . it's time to be movin on.

The rest of this book is about getting through. When we are strong enough to remember what has happened to us and to contemplate the implications of what has happened for the rest of our lives, we are awake in limbo and ready to move on.

3

Why Me?

I had a favorite nurse in the hospital. Among her many duties, she administered my tube feedings, patiently forcing green gunk down the plastic tube that ran through my nose into my stomach. Since I could not yet talk, I wrote her a note one evening: "I feel like a baby bird. You are my Momma bird, poking half-digested worms down my throat." She laughed; no one had ever said that before. I was an unusual patient, she said—in my will to live, my tolerance for pain, and my wild imagination. I also did not deserve my cancer. She wondered aloud that I had no risk factors: "Never smoked, hardly drank, and certainly didn't chew tobacco." We had many conversations, half-written, half-spoken, while she fed me. When I was free of the naso-gastric tube and ready for discharge, she came to say goodbye. "Let me give you a piece of advice. I've seen a lot of cancer patients," she explained. "Don't drive yourself crazy asking why this happened to you. It makes no sense. Enjoy your life. You truly know how precious it is."

GLENNA

My good nurse was right. We can drive ourselves crazy asking why. But I have never met a cancer patient, including myself, who could resist the temptation. In fact, there are two impossible questions that haunt those of us with cancer. The first is, Why me? to which there is seldom an answer. The more troubling question is, Will I die? to which the answer is absolute—yes. (Although, if we are lucky, we won't die from this cancer.) Since we don't want to face that answer, we focus on what we cannot know, Why me? Of course, if you are among the few cancer patients who know the probable cause of their cancers, then Why me? may not be a pressing question. Similarly, if you have a very strong family history for your cancer, then you may experience this issue differently.

Why Ask Why?

For many of us, asking Why me? is our first effort to reclaim our lives after we wake up in limbo. The need to understand why bad things happen to us seems to be nearly universal. Most patients create an explanation for their cancer. Having a personal theory does not help us live longer, and depending on the theory, it may not even make us feel better. However, not having a theory seems to make us feel worse. Creating an explanation allows us to make sense of a very threatening experience. And making sense of our lives helps us to go on, even in the face of danger.

So, against the advice of my wise and caring nurse, we are going to ask why. Not because we have the right answers, but because the need to ask is so strong, and the answers we create reveal so much about ourselves.

People who work with victims have noted that the injured are often full of self-doubt and self-blame. They replay the traumatic event (whether it was an earthquake, fire, war, rape, or illness) asking, "Why didn't I . . . ?" "What if . . . ?" And concluding, "If only . . ." To the observer, such self-recrimination seems both futile and cruel, but it also appears to be a necessary part of the process of coming to terms with trauma.

Most of us are invested in thinking of ourselves as survivors, not victims, of cancer. The word *victim* makes it sound as though we will die from our disease, while *survivors*, by definition, survive. However, any serious injury or illness is likely to leave us feeling weakened, confused, vulnerable—as if we, and/or the world, are out of whack. Nothing, including ourselves, seems quite what it used to be. This particular mix of thoughts and feelings is the essence of victimization *and* of waking up in limbo. Despite our determination to be more than victims, we have the classic symptoms, and we ask the classic question: Why me?

The Wish to Undo

Every victim wants to rewrite his or her story so it never really happened. Most of us feel this urge right from the start. We replay the moment of diagnosis over and over in our minds, hoping to change the words. Some cancer patients go from doctor to doctor, seeking not a second but a hundredth opinion, hoping to find someone who will say, "No. It's not cancer."

Although I never doubted my diagnosis, I had several friends who urged me to seek other opinions. One was my friend Louise, who is also a physician. She was chairing a meeting at which I was scheduled to speak. When I called to cancel, she expressed her concern and quickly moved on to discuss the program and other potential speakers. We said goodbye, and she wished me luck. Two minutes later, my phone rang. It was Louise. She said, "I'm sitting here in shock. This cannot be happening to you. I want you to get another pathologist to read your slides. I think they've made a mistake." And she launched into a mini biology lesson on the cell structure of viruses that look like my form of cancer. I was touched. The wish to undo bad news is so strong that even doctors want to reverse bad diagnoses.

People who love us often want to shield us from the unavoidable trauma of the diagnosis. Four years after her breast cancer was first diagnosed, Barbara remembers that when the biopsy confirmed a malignancy, she had trouble saying the word "cancer." Her sister said, "Every time you say the word 'cancer,' you start crying. Why don't you call it something else?" But Barbara knew that would not solve her problem. "I told my sister, 'I want to get to the point where I can say it. The more I say it, the less frightening it's going to become. I just need to work through this.'"

Other cancer patients try to undo their cancer after the fact. One cancer survivor told how she was startled to learn that some cancer patients insist that "it never happened," despite the evidence. As Charlotte was preparing for her chemotherapy, she remembered that "there was a woman in school who had cancer, and she had the most fabulous wig. I was anticipating a wig for my hair, and I had asked about it. I was told not to call her because she wouldn't talk about it, even with another cancer patient." Charlotte was appalled. "I think that's wrong. It's very important that you open up and talk." Although I share Charlotte's bias, I believe it is equally important to remember that we each deal with trauma in our own way. There have been times when I was neither ready nor willing to discuss my cancer with others. During the long first year after surgery, when my speech was badly impaired, I was not about to explain to the strangers who treated me like a drunk that I was, in fact, recovering from surgery for cancer.

Almost Forty Questions

Since most of us recognize that we cannot undo the fact that we have had cancer, we try to understand it. Understanding becomes a substitute for control; it is second best, but it's better than no control at all. If we can explain our cancer in a way that "guarantees" that it will not come back, so much the better.

Why me? is impossible to answer, in part, because it is many different questions rolled into one. It includes questions of science—and of sin. What have I done wrong? (A question of sin.) What have I done to deserve this? (A question of justice.) What are the known causes of this illness? (A medical question.) Why now? (A question of cause and effect.) How can I prevent a recurrence? (A question of medicine and of how to control one's destiny.) What does it mean? (A question arising from the human need for meaning.) And the Why? Why? Why? of the curious or furious child. All these questions are normal, legitimate, and common to survivors of trauma.

What Have I Done?

Our willingness to ask the question What have I done? says it all. Most of us will blame ourselves before we will entertain the possibility that we have limited control over our own lives. Our self-blame takes two forms, and the difference is subtle but important. We imagine that we have caused our cancer either by something we have done—or by something we have failed to do.

Although the notion that cancer is a punishment for our sins may remain unconscious or unspoken, it appears to be present in a surprising number of cancer patients and their family members. A recent study of Canadian children with cancer and their parents by David Bearison and his colleagues revealed that half of the adults blamed themselves for their child's cancer. (Only 20 percent of the children practiced self-blame.) What the parents blamed themselves for directly was a sin. They actually believed that their use of illicit drugs or their adultery had caused the child's cancer. The parents' reasoning defied medical science but reflected their belief that sin will be punished.

For many of us, the idea of cancer as a direct punishment for our sins is too antiscientific to believe. However, if we examine the causal theories we create, we may find sin lurking just below the surface of our reasoning. For example, women who are sexually active at an early age and have many sexual partners are, in fact, at higher risk for cervical cancer. Disentangling the "sin" (of "promiscuity") from the science (of statistical risk) in cervical cancer is difficult at best. Even if the form of cancer that we have does not appear directly linked to behavior that we feel guilty or ashamed about, we may, like the Canadian parents, nevertheless imagine it to be a retribution for our sins. Virginia, who had throat cancer thirty years ago and is now in her fifties, is a psychotherapist, so she was able to speak from her personal experience as well as her clinical observations. Although she did not believe that sin had played a part in her illness, she noted that "many people feel they're being punished for some wrongdoing."

If our theories include sex and drugs, or rock and roll (or anything else that we feel guilty about), we may need to reexamine our religious beliefs. When life gets tough, many of us fall back on the stern God of our childhood encounters with religion. We actually believe that bad things happen to bad people—even though we know better.

Even if we do not think that cancer is punishment for our sins, we may still prefer to believe that we have done something to deserve it—not a major sin, not gluttony or sloth, just bad eating or not enough exercise. If we can believe that we caused our own cancer, we maintain a sense of personal control. We can change the faulty behavior—if we can figure out what it was.

When we ask the What have I done? question, we are using self-blame to maintain our sense of justice. We have a powerful need to believe that life is somehow fair, that there is justice in this world. Psychologists have long known that people tend to blame the victims of misfortune. Even the victims blame themselves. Our primitive sense of justice is ruled by a cruel logic: if we want to believe that we will get what we deserve, then we must deserve what we get.

Barbara blamed her original breast cancer on faulty health habits and set out to correct those habits. She coped with getting cancer the first time by deciding to take more control of her life. "I was determined to do what I had to do to take control, get through it, get beyond it, and get on with a healthy life." But she could not justify her recurrence: "I thought, 'I did all the right things. How can it be back? This must be a mistake.'"

I remember the anger so many of my close friends felt when I had cancer. Since my compulsive health habits were a standing joke among them (who else flosses her teeth after every meal?), the injustice was all the more blatant. After years of teasing, I appreciated their sympathy, but I didn't share their outrage at the time. However, when my closest colleague had a major seizure this year, I was beside myself. By the time she was diagnosed, we were both relieved that it was epilepsy instead of a brain tumor. But while we waited, I was furious—like some crazed dragon, shedding tears and breathing fire. It was simply too awful and too unfair. She was in better physical condition than I had ever dreamed of being. Then I remembered her rage at my cancer; I felt that rage now for her.

Asking, "What have I done to deserve this?" barely masks the angry cry, "I don't deserve this!" And you don't. None of us deserves cancer.

What Are the Known Causes of Cancer?

There are a few known causes of cancer. A family history of the disease (genetic vulnerability), exposure to cancer causing agents (carcinogens) including tobacco and alcohol, several viruses, drug and radiation treatments, sun exposure, and dietary factors may contribute to certain cancers. But for Lisa and me and for most of you, the causes of our particular diseases are unknown. However, that doesn't stop us from building theories.

While cancer specialists are quick to say that the cause of most cancer is unknown, most patients believe that they know the cause of *their* cancers. A nationally renowned cancer specialist, Dr. Jimmie Holland of Memorial Sloan-Kettering Cancer Center, appreciates this difference in perspective and lets her patients know it: "I tell patients and their families, 'We don't know what causes cancer. We do know that when something bad happens, we all look for a reason or something to blame. So, we understand that you may feel differently from your doctors about this, and that's OK.'"

Patients need to know—or at least to believe that they do. In the Canadian study mentioned earlier, both parents and children felt better if they blamed an external cause (such as a test from God, an injury, or the environment). If they blamed themselves or found nothing to blame, they had more trouble coping. In a separate study of adult cancer victims, Dr. Shelley Taylor and her colleagues at UCLA Medical Center found that

95 percent of a group of women with breast cancer had private theories about why they had developed cancer. Are you curious about those theories? The most commonly cited cause was general stress. When a specific stressor was blamed, it was usually marital. After stress, the women cited exposure to carcinogens, then heredity, and finally poor diet or injuries to the breast. Unlike the results of the Canadian study, the results of this research did not show that believing in one cause was better than believing in another. The nature of the theory each woman held did not help her live longer nor improve her emotional adjustment. The need to find an explanation seemed to be an end in itself.

If You Have a Family History   Some people inherit a vulnerability to certain forms of cancer—it literally runs in the family. Yet if you believe that your family history predisposes you to cancer, take a closer look. Experts find that people frequently believe they are at greater risk than they actually are and that they blame heredity when it may not be the cause. Most cancers are not hereditary. Only 15 percent of the most common cancers are believed to have a hereditary component. If you have not already had genetic counseling, and you find yourself waiting for the "time bomb" to go off, seek cancer risk analysis from a qualified specialist.

Although we do not know all the links between heredity and cancer, we do know that patients with a family history often react to the diagnosis in a special way—they are almost relieved. These patients don't need to ask why, to them it seems only a question of when. If you expect to get cancer, then the initial diagnosis has less shock value. Dealing with the concrete reality of cancer is a relief from the endless anxiety of waiting. When the time bomb finally goes off, it may cause less damage than you had feared.

Charlotte had a strong family history of breast cancer. Both her mother and grandmother had died from the disease. Charlotte was in her mid forties when Lisa and I interviewed her, and her cancer had been diagnosed three years earlier. "I had been waiting," she said. "I had expected this since my grand-mother died when she was forty-nine. Then my mother died when she was forty-six." Because they had both died, Charlotte had always assumed that she would die too. Following a dou-ble mastectomy and seven months of chemotherapy, Charlotte had a hopeful prognosis, and her fear diminished: "Everything that I had dreaded all those years didn't come true." The worst had happened, and, so far, she had survived it.

However, once treatment is over, those of us with a family history of cancer face the same uncertain future as every other cancer survivor. We may not ask Why me? but our other ques-tions are just as real. And there is an additional, heavily loaded question: Will my fate be the same as my relative's? Charlotte's story illustrates the powerful effect of family history on our ex-pectations and perhaps our treatment choices.

Even after treatment, Charlotte admits, "I still worried that I was going to follow my mother." Charlotte dealt with this fear by emphasizing the differences in their stages of disease and types of treatment. "I separated myself from my mother, thinking that I can go this way and she went that way. We're different. It helped a lot." Although Charlotte doesn't say so directly, I suspect that her treatment choices were dictated, in part, by the fear of following in her mother's path. The first thing she said in her interview was, "I had a double mastec-tomy, one was therapeutic and one was prophylactic, because of my mother and my high risk. After that I had chemotherapy for seven months, and now I'm taking tamoxifen." Later, she explained that her mother had had a single mastectomy, and "then she got cancer in the other breast four years later, and she did not have chemotherapy." Although treatment recom-mendations change with time and new technology, Charlotte's thinking makes clear the importance to her of choosing a dif-ferent course of treatment in order to believe that she will have a different outcome.

Treatment decisions are often difficult even without a fam-ily history to complicate matters. What worked for a relative may not work for us, and a treatment that failed them may save us. Because cancer treatment is a rapidly evolving area of medicine, there may have been *no* effective treatment available to many of our ancestors. Treatment decisions must be made on an individual basis in consultation with experts. However, it is naïve to ignore the effect of our family history—on our risk of cancer *and* on our expectations.

Further Complications from Family History   In all areas of life, our worst fears and fondest dreams are shaped by our early experiences within our families. Cancer is no exception. If family members have survived cancer, we have role models of survival that may give us hope. If family members have died of cancer, we may, like Charlotte, expect the worst. But it is more than the medical history that shapes our expectations, it is the social history as well. How did our families deal with the illness?

Many of the survivors interviewed spontaneously related stories about the illnesses of family members and friends, indicating that these associations are present in all of us and constantly shaping our experiences. I have several memories of cancer from childhood, including my dreadful grandmother preparing for bed, taking off the biggest bra I had ever seen. There was her chest, a hollow of rippling scars with a huge, pendulous breast to one side. I was three, and even then I didn't hate her for looking strange. I hated her because she didn't like children, and that meant me. When Nama was around, I was to be seen, not heard, and seen only at her request.

Three years later, my favorite aunt lay on a cot in a darkened room, a woman faith healer standing over her. When the healer noticed me, she pulled a curtain, and my aunt disappeared from view. Aunt Gustie had cervical cancer, but had refused surgery. In 1953, her diagnosis was just big words to me. Years later, I would understand that she was part of the first wave of American women whose cancer, detected by a pap smear, could be cured. But nothing in Gustie's experience prepared her to believe in a cure. My mother was a nurse by training, and I remember her rage at my aunt for rejecting the newest and best in medical care. I also remember my uncle, who loved his wife, sitting in his recliner chair, sobbing. My mother was insisting that Aunt Gustie get proper care; Uncle Jack was choking out phrases: "But she won't"; "I can't stand to lose her"; "But, Mary, what can I do?" My mother, feeling as helpless to change the course of events as my uncle, gave up the argument. And so it happened that as a six-year-old, I was the companion my aunt took to that faith healer's "clinic" in a farmhouse in the country.

Those early experiences affect me to this day. My grandmother was badly scarred, but she was alive and mean and unashamed of her wound. My beloved aunt died when I was seven. When my cancer was diagnosed, I chose surgery without a second thought, but I also know that people I love have made and will make very different choices than I would make, and like my uncle, I struggle to respect those choices.

For those of us who have had cancer and those who love us, it is worthwhile to ask: In what ways are our expectations influenced by earlier family experiences? Here are some specific questions that may bring more memories to light. Who was sick in your family? What did you think about that person? How did other family members relate to him or her? What about your friends at school? Did any of them experience serious illnesses? Did any of them die? Name those associations. Talking about them will not make bad things happen, and saying them out loud may help you understand seemingly irrational feelings and fears. It can also help you understand why others react in ways that take you by surprise.

To illustrate the usefulness of sharing memories with one's current family and friends, let me tell you about my husband's early experience. Curtis has no family history of cancer; instead, both his mother and maternal grandmother were world-class hypochondriacs. Consequently, he has never been sympathetic or patient with illness, including his own. The early "illnesses" in his family deprived him of too much nurturing and care.

When my cancer was diagnosed and the surgery had been fully explained to us, it was clear that I would be completely incapacitated for several weeks. As we drove home from the doctor's office, my husband said, "This is going to be a real challenge for me. I know that your cancer is real, and this surgery is absolutely necessary. You aren't anything like my mother or my grandmother, but I'm afraid that I'll pull away from you, just as I did with them."

To his credit, he did not withdraw, but it was hard. He wanted me up and well far sooner than I had the strength. He brought a set of hand and leg weights to my hospital room so I could exercise in bed, and when I got home, I found a new exercise unit in the guest room. He wanted me strong and active, and so did I, but at the time, I didn't know whether to laugh or cry. Because we both understood what was going on, we were able to laugh *and* cry. And I still use that exercise equipment.

Why Now?

On the face of it, Why now? is a ludicrous question. As if another time would be more convenient. Couldn't we just reschedule? Or better yet, cancel the appointment? Such wishful thinking aside, this question is tied to the deeper issues of justice and control and to our need for a cause. Now may be the "wrong" time because we have done nothing to deserve this cancer—recently. Or we may think that we could handle the situation more ably at another time. Finally, if we believe in the law of cause and effect, then we search the time preceding our diagnosis for the cause of our illness.

Like every cancer patient I have ever met, I too searched for an explanation. Among my private theories, I entertained the possibility that my demanding and sometimes chaotic work travel had worn me down, body and spirit, thus leaving me vulnerable to an errant cell. In the year preceding my diagnosis, I frequently woke in the night in a strange bed, room, hotel, and city. I often joked that the worst part of being so disoriented was finding my way to the bathroom. After I got cancer, I thought maybe those mysterious bathrooms had not been the worst part. I decided that feeling so deeply torn between conflicting responsibilities at work and at home had not been good for me, and I decided to make some changes. At least, I would be happier in my life, and who knows, maybe I would live longer.

Lisa also searched the time preceding her diagnosis for possible causes. She said, "I'd finally finished my doctoral dissertation, and I felt a loss of purpose, a real letdown. I was depressed for quite a while, and I believe that the stress of that time contributed to my cancer." However, Lisa then carried her thinking about this belief further: "There's a really superstitious element to this kind of thinking. If I don't pay attention to these very quiet thoughts, I can believe that completing any major project puts me at risk of death."

Even patients like Charlotte, who can identify a scientifically accepted cause for their disease, tend to look at the time preceding diagnosis for additional clues. Charlotte summarized a stressful period for the school board on which she served as "something that started slowly, and it grew and gathered momentum, and then it exploded in my cancer." Although she went on to say that the situation had not caused her cancer, she could not help noting that "the timing was just then." We think if we can figure out the answer to Why now? then we may be able to prevent our cancer from happening again—which is our next question.

How Can I Prevent a Recurrence?

The question How can I prevent a recurrence? is clearly linked to known causes and cures. But it is also more than a medical question. Our deeper motives are apparent in our tendencies as cancer patients to believe in personally controllable causes, despite medical evidence to the contrary. Apparently, we need to restore our sense of control more than we need accurate medical information. One of the cancer patients interviewed by Shelley Taylor explained her reasoning this way: "I looked over the known causes of cancer—like viruses, radiation, genetic mutations, environmental carcinogens—and the one I focused on very strongly was diet. I know now why I focused on it. It was the only one that was simple enough for me to understand

and change. You eat something that's bad for you, you get sick." By selecting a cause over which she had control, she believed that she could control her cancer.

We hope to prevent a recurrence by choosing a cause over which we have control or one which is no longer in effect. If the stress is past (the bad marriage is over, the bad boss is history), then by the logic of cause and effect, we believe that we are safe. We may not need to focus on a specific cause in order to believe that we can protect ourselves from a recurrence. Bente is a spiritual consultant who developed invasive cervical cancer when she was fifty. Bente's general beliefs about the psychic roots of disease allow her to feel safe from a recurrence because she has experienced a spiritual shift since her cancer: "I don't believe something can reoccur, if you've changed," she said. She has suffered enough misfortune in her life to know that something else may happen, and it may be bad, but it will not be a repetition of past misfortune because she has moved beyond that.

What Is the Meaning of This?

Of all the variations on Why me? the most profound and enduring is What is the meaning of this? Most survivors create meaning from the unfortunate experience of cancer, so that over time, the thrust of our questions shifts. We ask: How can I learn and grow from this experience? What good can come of this? If this approach sounds a little too good to be true, listen to how other survivors see it. When we asked Virginia if she ever asked herself Why me? she said, "Of course! You're talking to a psychologist! [Although it's] not so much 'Why me?' as if I've been singled out. I don't have that sense at all. For me, it's more a question of 'What does this experience say about me?' or 'What meaning do I derive from it?'" In fact, Virginia has derived great meaning from having had cancer at an early age. Her questions about the meaning of life's events led her to a career in psychology, and later scares of recurrence have consistently moved her to deeper levels of self-exploration.

Similarly, Judy spoke of using her cancer experiences to further her personal growth. Like Virginia, Judy explained that she had never asked, "Why me and not someone else?" Instead, she had raged, "Why? Why? Why?" Like Job in the biblical tale, Judy railed at the universe, and then made her peace with the injustice in a way that preserves her faith in herself and in larger forces: "Over time, I've developed an understanding of the role of breast cancer in my life that satisfies my need for personal growth."

Bente also saw cervical cancer as an opportunity: "In a way it pulled together all my life lessons. . . . It was an intensification of energy that could push me through." After she had answered Why me? in a highly personal way, she asked herself another series of questions: "How do we nourish ourselves?" "How are we nourished by the people in our lives?" "Do they allow us to nourish them?" The questions were about love as an act of giving and receiving. "The lesson came back to choosing myself, and knowing that that's not selfish."

Brian has also wanted something good to come of his painful experience. Brian is a geologist in his forties, who was happily married and had two young sons when a melanoma on his back was diagnosed six years ago. In talking with him, it is clear that both his well-trained scientific mind and his dry sense of humor have served him well. With characteristic wit, he says that when he was first diagnosed, he considered "becoming the Melanoma Poster Boy, warning all who would listen about the importance of protection from ionizing radiation and the great advantage of early detection." But he settled on a sober task that could benefit him and those he loves: "For me, melanoma could be a blessing in disguise, an opportunity to deal with all the issues surrounding my own mortality." Then he brought that grand plan right down to earth: "It's a clear challenge to get my shit together."

The Importance of Self-Pity

Why me? is also a plaintive cry of self-pity disguised as a question. Feeling sorry for ourselves is a natural reaction when something terrible happens. Unfortunately, self-pity is not a presentable emotion in most social circles. We do not approve of it in ourselves or others, and hence, we hide the feeling behind a screen of intelligent questions. How much simpler it would be to say, "I feel so sad and sorry *for myself* that this has happened." If we are sensitive and caring people, we are able to extend such compassion to others, yet we often withhold it from ourselves.

Charlotte talked about the special comfort one of her friends was able to give. While she was still in the hospital recovering from a double mastectomy with immediate reconstruction, many friends came by to offer reassurance and good cheer. They told her how strong she was, how surely she would beat this cancer. In effect, they discounted her physical and emotional agony, and minimized her risk. In contrast, another friend sat with Charlotte, massaging her shoulders and saying, "This is shit! Why does this happen?" Charlotte recognized that her friend was saying, " 'I feel so sorry for you,' but she said it in her way." It was deeply affirming and such a relief to have someone feel sorry for her when she was feeling sorry for herself.

When self-pity becomes a habit, it becomes even less attractive, to be sure, and no longer stirs the compassion of others. But there are times when a deep sadness at the human condition and our part in it is right on the mark. Having cancer is one of those times. Chapter Five, about survivor grief, explains that process in greater detail.

There are many ways to recognize our sorrow and honor it. We can, for one thing, talk and cry with people who love us and truly understand. It is critically important, however, that we share these feelings with people who can tolerate the pain—those who will neither judge us weak nor try to talk us out of how we feel. Charlotte was very sensitive to the fact that the well-meaning friends who minimized her plight could not help her, and she explained this with the perfect analogy of the "child who's been out bicycle riding and comes in screaming because he fell and cut his knee. If you say to that child, 'It's nothing. What are you crying for?' [it doesn't help]. Instead, you take the child in your lap, and you kiss and boo hoo, and you say, 'Oh, I know it hurts, and I hope it feels better.' There's such a difference."

Another way to express genuine self-pity is through ceremony. Most of us use ritual and ceremony to mark important events and feelings. That is what holiday and anniversary celebrations are supposed to be about; unfortunately, that meaning is often lost. In our private ceremonies, we embody the deepest meanings of events in our life. Such acts are often simple, even childlike. On the night before my admission to the hospital, my husband and I drove to a lake near our home. We sat on the grass, watching the sun set, and cried together. We did not know what the surgery would reveal: had the cancer spread into my jaw or lymph nodes? Would I have enough of my tongue to speak again? Would I have my face?

As the blood-orange sun disappeared and the sky faded through mauves to the twilight gray I've loved since childhood, I made my wishes on the first night star. I had not done that since childhood. Similarly, I have friends who lit candles for me during my hospitalization and later when I had scares of recurrence. Those simple rituals, often carried over from childhood, can give great comfort.

The most powerful ceremony I have ever experienced was one my husband performed for my birthday, when I came home from the hospital. Curtis was raised in the Primitive Baptist Church, in which foot washing is the primary sacrament. He invited our closest friends and family for a healing ceremony. First, he offered us bread in a beautiful handmade enamel bowl with a blue candle burning in the center. He said that the bread, as the staff of life, was symbolic of enriching the everyday necessities so that they bring joy. We toasted my health and the love amongst us with champagne. Then Curtis returned with the bowl full of water, and I realized that he was going to wash my feet. As he knelt, he thanked the Lord of life and death for not taking me from him and asked that he be an agent of my healing. Then he dried my feet. In that ritual of humility, he contained the sorrow he felt for himself at the prospect of losing me and reminded all of us that self-pity can be elegant in its honesty.

Our Questions Serve a Deeper Purpose

The litany of questions that we ask puts distance between us and the painful experience of surviving treatment only to wake up in limbo. Remember being told something you did not want to hear as a child and arguing, "But why? Why? Why?" If we could stall long enough, maybe the inevitable would just go away. Similarly, the endless questions we ask about our cancer allow us an emotional stall at a time when slowing down the pace of events and feelings is probably a very good idea. Diagnosis and treatment happen way too fast.

Even before the diagnosis is formal, our minds are racing. Barbara remembers going in for a routine mammogram. The nurse who examined her first detected a suspicious lump, and within minutes, she had had the mammogram. As Barbara puts it, "Essentially, you just felt fine, now you might have cancer, and you might die. Suddenly, you're wondering who's going to come to your funeral, and you don't even know if you have a malignancy."

By the end of the day, Barbara had seen two specialists and had a biopsy scheduled for the following day. She remembers, "I drove home crying, and I thought, 'Oh, it's funny how a day just sort of flip-flops.'" Flip-flop, indeed! With definitive diagnosis, our lives shift into fast-forward. Prompt treatment offers our best hope for survival, so it's full speed ahead. Within one week, Barbara had surgery and was scheduled for radiation. For most cancer patients, things do not slow down until treatment is complete.

Our questions are an intellectual detour that slows down the rush of feelings and restarts our thought processes, which may have been overwhelmed by the raw fear of death. Although we may seem to be harassing ourselves with unanswerable questions, in fact there is a method to our madness.

Our intellectualizing reduces intolerable anxiety and allows us to move at our own pace toward a painful conclusion. The dreaded conclusion is not only death, but the death of our illusion of immortality.

When to Stop Asking

Why me? is often our first question, and the lament behind it, in all its complexity, persists. Years after diagnosis and treatment, we may find ourselves revising our theories. The question simply cannot be put to rest. It is unanswerable, yet (perhaps therefore) it will not go away. A reexamination of the question may be triggered by a fear of recurrence, another illness or injury, the diagnosis of a friend or family member, normal aging changes, or who knows what. A preoccupation with that question and all its subsequent questions delays our acceptance of the real conditions of our life. At some point, we must set the questions aside and get on with life.

Reynolds Price, the gifted writer and a survivor of spinal cancer, offers an answer that is an ultimate answer for some: "Some vital impulse spared my needing to reiterate the world's most frequent and pointless question in the face of disaster— *Why? Why me?* I never asked it; the only answer is, of course, *Why not?*" This line of thinking spared Price the need to question. However, for other survivors, the answer Why not? offers no closure. It is another trap, this one filled with guilt.

Survivor Guilt

A major barrier to getting on with life after a traumatic event is guilt. Many of the Why me? questions contain elements of guilt, but there is another potential source of guilt, the fact of survival. Getting a cure—what we most want and have endured the miseries of treatment to attain—may generate a new set of doubts and questions.

Guilt among the survivors of traumatic experiences is so common that it has a name, survivor guilt, and is well documented in the literature on survivors. (A useful discussion of survivor guilt can be found in the book *Human Adaptation to Extreme Stress*.) The question we ask is, Why have I lived when others die? We may feel unworthy of our good fortune. News of someone else's death from "our disease" not only stirs our fear of dying, it calls up guilt—for living. In the strange equation in our mind, our life is linked to the other's death. There is powerful word magic in the Christian tradition that may set people up for the irrational belief that good fortune comes at the expense of another being. But "He died that we might live" applies to Christ, not other cancer victims. It is cancer that kills others, not our living.

Some survivors even feel guilty when their treatment is less horrific than they had expected or than the treatment others must endure. Initially, Barbara had a lumpectomy and radiation. "I thought I'd gotten off really easy. I felt guilty. I thought, 'Here I am. I've had cancer, but it was a simple operation. I've had radiation, but I'm really okay.'" Then she dreamed that she could see inside her breast, which contained a yellow raspberry. That raspberry represented all her doubts about the cure and her fears of a recurrence. "I realized that I hadn't gotten away easy—the fear never goes away. No one really gets off easy."

In order to survive our guilt, we need to tell our story—over and over and over again. And we need an attentive and sympathetic audience. Our family and friends may grow weary of these repeat performances, but we need to trust our inner urge to tell it all yet again. Cancer support groups and therapists know the importance of this repetition. We all need to retell our story until we have worn the shock and the shame out of it. Writing the story may help, recounting every detail. Brian, who wrote the story of his cancer in seventeen terse and witty pages, said that the act of writing finally released him from much of the anger he had felt. However we choose to do it, telling the story as many times as *we* need to is essential to our recovery.

I learned the importance of both repetition and mundane detail in my own psychoanalysis. I began analysis nine months after my cancer surgery. It had been a dream since college, but I had never had the time or the money for such an undertaking. Those limitations had protected me from deeper doubts: did I really have the strength of character and the courage to face my demons? Having faced my death, I thought I did. I had also hit the emotional bottom of my limbo, and I was no longer too proud to ask for help. At one particularly frustrating point in my analysis, I was moaning to my analyst about how slow the process was, and how slow I was to change: "I've dealt with this same material [not cancer] so many times that I'm boring myself to death. I feel like an old dog with no new tricks, circling the same damn bush in the same old yard, peeing in the same old place." Then I begged, "How many more times do I have to do this?" My analyst chuckled, "Oh, maybe only a few hundred."

In addition to doing things to help ourselves, if we feel the need, we can do something for others who are less fortunate. Many cancer survivors work as volunteers with patient advocacy groups (see the Resources for some of these groups). Although we have done nothing for which we need to make amends, "good deeds" can make us feel better. Beyond allowing us to feel atonement, such activities can add positive meaning to our lives. They also help us shift our focus from the meaning of our cancer to the larger meaning of our life.

The good fortune to survive may instill in us a special sense of purpose. Why have I been spared? can be answered in many ways, and those answers may give new meaning to our lives. We do not need to *read meaning into* the random events of life or romanticize our bad fortune. But we can *create meaning out of* an unfortunate experience. Having escaped death, for a time, we can make that time count. That is exactly what most of the survivors Lisa and I quote in these pages chose to do, and it is part of our motive for writing this book. The writing has allowed us to tell our stories yet again and to shape them so that they may be of use to others.

One of the men we interviewed is an artist and a teacher in his fifties. Bill had Hodgkin's disease twelve years ago. As an artist, his stock-in-trade is the creative expression of his deepest concerns. Bill painted prolifically throughout his radiation treatments. During that time, he painted his first image of death and the beyond, and this motif continues to emerge in his work. On the day before his interview, he had given the students in his painting class a particularly difficult assignment, and he reported:

At the beginning of the day, they thought, "Oh, my god! What has he done to us now?" At the end of the day, they had all been able to do it, partially carried by my confidence in their ability. The lesson, and the lesson in all of my teaching, is that you can do more than you think you can. So, if someone is going through the cancer experience thinking, "Why me? Poor me. How am I going to get through this?" it's really an opportunity to see how much you can do, how much there is inside you. We are all so far from using our full potential that cancer is an opportunity to see that there is that potential."

Illness often requires strengths of character we did not know we possessed. It also prompts magical thinking our rational minds would deny in a minute. As I was working on this chapter, I tore the cartilage and ligament in my right knee. "Why me? Why now?" I worried. A friend called in sympathy. "I can't believe that this has happened to you. Your legs are so strong," he moaned—knowing (in part) that if I could suffer such an unjust injury so could he. I was embarrassed to admit that I believed the same thing, that "this should not be happening to me! I'm too fit, too careful." As if illness and injury should make sense. Sometimes they do. But I, of all people, know better. Yet my craziness was not self-limiting. As I recovered from surgery, I literally heard a small voice in my head saying, "Oh, please, let me dance again. I'll be such a good girl. I'll do anything, just let me dance." I was bargaining. Caught in the act. Agh! This stuff is real, and knowing better is no protection.

4

Taking the First Steps: Fears of Recurrence

In a regular checkup, my doctor found a lump that he wanted my surgeon to check out. Since I couldn't get an appointment until the next week, I tried pushing aside my fear: it's nothing; don't jump to conclusions; surely I'm all right. But then I caught myself wondering what it would be like to die, how I would feel, what I would do. In this frame of mind, I went to see the movie Philadelphia. *In the theater, I finally cried as the hero came closer to his death, and when I left, I was still crying. As I drove home, I was consumed with thoughts of death. In my mind, I became the movie's hero in that hospital bed, struggling to breathe, my friends whispering around me. Then it hit me from my gut: wait a minute—I'm not sick; I'm not in that hospital bed; I can eat and make love and see the stars and hear the river. Even if I find out that I've had a recurrence, I'm here now, and I can be alive now. I felt an immediate and enormous relief and joy.*

LISA

I had never felt so aware of being alive. Afterward, I thought a lot about that moment, the abrupt shift from being consumed with fear of death to a sharp awareness of the simple and miraculous moments of being alive. To be strong enough to walk up a hill and smell the air as it came in from the ocean. To talk about inconsequential things with friends

61

and laugh. To have an appetite and be able to eat enough to satisfy my hunger and to taste the food I was eating. I was grateful for things I had always taken for granted.

This was a nearly magical transformation for me. For years, I had tried to will myself to appreciate being in the moment rather than replaying the past or worrying about the future. Staying in the here and now always felt like a homework assignment I couldn't quite master. And then, in the midst of real fear about my health, I suddenly felt alive, caught up in the present moment. Deep in my gut, I accepted that I can do nothing to change the fact that I will die sooner or later, like it or not, ready or not. What I can do is experience fully the other side of that terrible knowledge: I am alive now, and it feels wonderful.

Now that some time has passed, I also believe that focusing on being alive was an excellent defense mechanism. It was an instinctive way to comfort myself when thoughts of death were too close. Managing our fears of recurrence is a delicate balancing act, and it takes practice. We must somehow maintain an optimistic belief in our future yet not deny that death will come one day. It takes courage to plan for a future that still feels uncertain.

Fears of recurrence do not typically emerge until well after treatment has ended. Then a blanket of jumbled feelings smothers our former sense of well-being. I described this earlier as feeling as if someone had melted cheese over my brain. My vision seemed blurred; my head felt muffled. Disorientation, depression, confusion, and a vague uneasiness permeated me.

During recuperation from the trauma we have been through, we are too exhausted to cope with the big questions that were raised by our cancer and that are still lurking just behind the door. For the moment, as we are recovering, the door has to stay closed. But holding it closed begins to wear us out.

My exhaustion during this time was most apparent at work. If I knew what tasks and projects had to be done ahead of time, I was okay. But every time someone asked me to take responsibility for *anything* that was not on my list, no matter how small, I went into a panic. I fearfully believed that my energy was finite, that I was fragile and could lose control at any moment. I think that I was using most of my energy to keep that psychological door shut on the fears about cancer that were beginning to push to get out.

Over time, we regain some equilibrium; maybe it is just repeating the rituals of daily life that eventually brings us through the exhaustion and sense of blurred unreality. It was at this point that I began to feel assaulted by fear. Once we are awake and conscious that we are in limbo, we can begin to experience our fears of recurrence directly. If we are going to learn to move and later to dance in this strange new land, we must first find a balance between our hopes and our fears. This is much like learning to walk for the first time. We have to take it slowly, be gentle with ourselves when we fall down, and pick ourselves up repeatedly, lest we get stuck in limbo. We want to be dancing; we do not want to be stuck.

My depression lifted to reveal swarms of fears that my cancer would return. I had gained enough strength and distance from being sick to begin to let in the implications: I had been stripped of the belief that I was immortal. Fears of recurrence are brief reenactments of our recent cancer and painful reminders of our new understanding of mortality. These fears are little rips in the comforting denial of death that makes it possible for human beings to live relatively free of anxiety, to create lives that feel full and meaningful even in the face of eventual death.

Every ache, every wheeze, every bubble of gas I had foretold rampant unseen tumors. Sometimes I was able to see the humor in my obsession with my body, but only with the help of others and not very often. People in my support group were particularly helpful, as was Glenna. Anyone who has had cancer understands the phenomenon of this kind of worry. Mentioning it to someone who has "been there" often provides instant relief, even through something as simple as a smile of shared recognition. I had particularly rich soil in which my fears could grow, since melanoma is notoriously unpredictable and can show up in any organ of the body at any time; recurrences sometimes take place as long as twenty years after the original site has been treated.

The Fears Change but Never End

Every survivor we interviewed, even the ones whose cancer was twenty or thirty years ago, was still vulnerable to fears that his or her cancer had recurred. Certain events will make fears flare up—hearing of the death of a friend, reading an article about cancer, developing a mysterious symptom, having a regularly scheduled physical checkup. It happens to all of us.

The act of writing this book and especially this chapter triggered cancer anxieties in me. In order to write in a way that would be meaningful and helpful to readers, Glenna and I had to be willing to reexperience our cancers from the time of diagnosis to right now. We learned very soon that we had great resistance to doing this. In no way did I want to physically remember the horrible, intense, consuming, hopeless anxiety of those early days. For nearly a year after treatment, I was either overwhelmed with terror and hopelessness or fighting off those feelings. It was a dark time for me, and it is hard to revisit.

We will always be vulnerable to fearing our cancer may return. But we are more fearful in the first year or two after recovery, which is also when we are at highest risk.

Ann, in her second year of recovery from a metastasis of her melanoma to her lymph system, thought her worst nightmare had come to pass once. Why not again? She found (along with many others) that she was most vulnerable to her fears at night.

I've been successful at pushing this back up to a point. I'm successful until I get into bed at night. Unless I'm totally exhausted, I find that I seem to go inside myself and think about it. . . . I start thinking that I should write out my autobiography so that my kids have it or the grandchildren will have it. . . . You start cleaning out your house, going through drawers and tossing out stuff you've been saving for years and you don't need any more. You kind of wind up. But as [my husband] said, "As long as you have something to clean up, you can't die."

Barbara is the survivor who had a lumpectomy and a subsequent double mastectomy. Fears of recurrence are so powerful that even when both breasts were gone, Barbara was afraid.

After the first surgery, my thoughts were just, "How will I know if it's happening again? If I get a cold, does that mean my immune system's down and I've got cancer somewhere in my body? If I have a headache, is it a brain tumor? If my leg hurts or my hip hurts, is it in my bones?" It was the insecurity of wondering if it was going to come back, and how could I trust my body to let me know it was there. If I waited too long, was it going to spread all over my body? . . . I don't trust it yet. I know that it's supposed to be gone, . . . but the uncertainty is still there.

Twelve years after her surgery for melanoma, Ellen has come to accept that although her cancer doesn't dominate her life as it once did, it will always be there. "When you live your life as a cancer survivor, you don't know. You don't know what your path is going to be. You just know you can do your best. . . . The part that's really hard to communicate to someone who isn't a cancer survivor is that on a day-to-day, moment-to-moment basis, you live with the fact that there may be [cancer] cells running around, that time bomb notion that there may be some cells on the loose; and if it's not conscious, it's subconscious, but it's there. It's there all the time."

Even many years after successful treatment, an unexplained physical symptom can bring back fear of recurrence in the snap of a finger. Several months before Virginia's interview, she developed symptoms that alarmed both her and her physician, despite the fact that her throat cancer had been thirty years before. "I kept running into walls and stumbling and falling, and so finally my internist said, 'You need to go to a neurologist. We need to do an MRI and a CAT scan because it's possible you have a brain tumor.' . . . It turned out I had an inner-ear virus. But what's interesting is that any time I stumble or any time something occurs now, I immediately leap to thinking it's cancer."

Neil's testicular cancer was twenty years ago, and he also recalled a recent scare:

> The thought of is it flu or is it cancer again receded at about the five-year marker. But I just went to get my eyes checked, and the doctor says, "Well, there's a spot on your retina." And he says, "Because of your history, we should follow this up because it could be a metastasis." . . . That freaked me out. Luckily, I was examined twenty minutes later by my surgeon down the hall, who said, "It's a freckle, and we'll watch it." But because this is the twentieth anniversary, and I'm ready to celebrate, to feel that worry again . . . was a real pain in the ass.

As Neil, a fifty-one-year-old psychologist, pointed out, the strength of the fear does diminish over time. We must learn how to listen to our bodies and interpret their signals correctly.

Signals from Within, or Am I Turning Into a Hypochondriac?

Most of us have two somewhat conflicting responses to our bodies. On the one hand, we feel deep distrust because they have betrayed us by allowing cancer cells to grow. We can't see inside ourselves to know whether and when those cells may decide to reappear and start munching away at us. On the other hand, when these cells were growing, our bodies also told us that something was really wrong. This happened to me twice.

For a long time, I had been meaning to see a dermatologist about some facial acne. It wasn't awful enough for me to drop everything for an appointment, but seeing zits appear at my age was demoralizing. I got a recommendation, and I carried the name of the doctor around in my pouch of notes and reminders. One day I just picked up the phone and made an appointment. The morning of my appointment, in the shower, I felt a little bump on my back. When I looked at it in the mirror, I saw that the bump was on a mole I had had all my life. After the doctor had checked my face and given me a prescription for Retin-A, he asked if there was anything else. I said, "Oh, could you just look at the mole on my back"—a request that saved my life. It was a brand-new melanoma, so thin it was barely there. The dermatologist removed it that day, I had follow-up surgery to clip away more skin to be sure no cancer cells had begun to stray out, and everyone thought that was that.

Two years later, my appetite decreased, and I felt slightly queasy when I ate. I started joking with my friends that I must have stomach cancer. After about two weeks of this, something clicked in my brain. I actually *listened* to what I had been saying, and I remembered my doctor's warning to pay attention to *any* physical change, anything out of the ordinary, and to check it out. So feeling a bit foolish about making such a fuss over an upset stomach, I went to my doctor, who found an enlarged lymph node under my arm. My melanoma had moved into my lymph system.

In this instance, I choose to believe that my body was telling me something was wrong, and I am thankful that I heard what it was saying. However, at other times, I have had worries that turned out to be nothing: lymph nodes that felt bigger than usual, asthma I was sure meant lung tumors. If you are not sure what your body is telling you, go to a physician who can evaluate your situation. I have also asked my friends to help me "listen" to what I am saying, in case I'm not hearing my own message. I had symptoms for over a month before I began talking about stomach cancer. It scares me to think what the consequences would have been if I had ignored my own words.

Jeannette, the retired professor, had an experience similar to mine when her cancer was first detected four years ago. In her interview, she reported:

My lung cancer was a very accidental discovery that probably would have occurred much later if it weren't for the nature of some symptoms which had, as it happens, nothing to do with the cancer. It was a chest symptom, kind of a grabby feeling, and it was kind of annoying and it persisted for several weeks so I couldn't attribute it to indigestion or anything like that. So I went to the doctor and got a chest x-ray . . . and the radiologist didn't like the way the x-ray looked. There were some suspicious signs. . . . [The doctors] finally decided it was cancer.

Distinguishing Symptoms from Fears

The trick is to read the signals correctly. And once we have had cancer, that turns out to be a nearly impossible task. If something has triggered our fear, one normal response is to express the fear as a physical symptom. Then we interpret the symptom as evidence of cancer. We may worry constantly about moles, colds, allergies, fatigue, or headaches and convince ourselves they are signs of cancer.

Katharine, a writer in her forties who recently survived cervical cancer, got news within one week that two of her childhood friends had died of cancer. This was more than a reminder of mortality; it was a bludgeon. Because her anxiety was too strong for her to tolerate, she unconsciously transformed it into a physical symptom. "My stomach became very distended, and when I ate, I felt too full. I convinced myself that I had tumors in my abdomen that were pressing on my stomach. My doctor checked everything and said I was fine, but I didn't believe him. I was dimly aware of thinking, at some level, 'If my friends can die, so can I.' Eventually, I started to burp like crazy, and my tummy went back to normal. It was like having a hysterical pregnancy or something."

This bloating was, in fact, an elegant metaphoric expression of the overwhelming (bloated) thoughts she had swallowed but was unable to express fully.

It may be comforting to remember that even those who have not had cancer have fearful fantasies about small symptoms. Writer Anne Lamott is sensitive to fears of cancer because of the deaths of her father from a brain tumor and of her best friend Pammy from breast cancer. She captures one of these painful moments and turns it into humor.

> Being a writer guarantees that you will spend too much time alone—and that as a result, your mind will begin to warp. . . . You'll notice a tiny mouth sore, one of those tiny canker sores that your tongue can't keep away from, that feels like a wound the size of a marble, but when you go to study it in the mirror, you see that it is a white spot roughly as big as a pinhead. Still, the next thing you know—because you are spending *too much time alone*—you are convinced that you have mouth cancer, just like good old Sigmund, and you know instantly that doctors will have to cut away half of your jaw, trying to save your miserable obsessive-compulsive head from being cannibalized by the cancer, and you'll have to go around wearing a hood over your entire face, and no one will ever want to kiss you again, not that they ever did.

Lamott is aware that her fantasies appear because she is alone a lot, and she recommends that writers call friends during their writing time to stay in touch with reality. This is not bad advice for all of us, even if we are not writers. I have found that hearing other people's stories gives me relief and a sense that I am not alone. There is another tip implied here. Writing out our fears in all their glory, even using humor when we can, may help us to shrink them back into manageable proportion.

Checking It Out

The bottom line, however, when we are getting signals from within, is that we check them out with our doctors and not worry that someone might think we are hypochondriacs. We should never sit alone with anxiety. Never shove fear under the rug and regret it later. Check it out.

In addition, regular physical checkups—particularly in the first several years after your cancer—are important for your peace of mind and to ensure early detection of any recurrence. Some people believe that the return of cancer will be signalled by pain or sickness. Sometimes it is, but frequently an early recurrence is silent. Often, your doctor will advise you to have physicals at appropriate intervals.

Regular physicals give some structure to the limbo of uncertainty we entered when our treatment was finished. In the first year after my surgery, I saw my surgeon, my dermatologist, and my internist every three months. I scheduled the appointments so that I saw one of them every month. Although the appointments raised some anxiety in me, they also provided me with reality checks and reassurance. At the end of the first year, my surgeon said he no longer needed to see me. I had mixed feelings of apprehension ("one less person to make sure I am healthy") and pride ("he believes I'm going to be fine"). I continue to see my dermatologist and my internist, but my appointments are less frequent. My vigilance is still high, but my dread of finding a problem has diminished.

Regular checkups also help to break down time into manageable chunks. Brian, the melanoma survivor who has been clear of his cancer for five years, said that at first he was sure it would return. Because it was too overwhelming for him to worry about unlimited years of uncertainty, he made a deal with himself to look ahead only to the next physical, three months away. This he could tolerate.

Regression in the Face of Fear

Fears of recurrence happen to all of us, and certain things can trigger those fears. I have discussed handling anxiety by consulting a physician, by talking to friends, and by using humor and writing. But what about the emotional ways we cope with fear?

One response many of us have is to regress. Regression is reverting to thoughts, feelings, and behaviors that we used at a much earlier age. Sometimes we regress when our more mature defenses are overwhelmed and stop functioning. This can easily happen with the simultaneous appearance of our fear of recurrence and our sense of powerlessness to alter reality. Regression is our automatic attempt to find peace and tranquility in the face of great stress. It is like the kindergartner who reverts to thumb-sucking when facing school for the first time.

Our vulnerability to cancer and death fears is too much like being children, when we had few skills and were dependent on others to take care of us. When we feel this vulnerable as adults, we may automatically regress. These are the times when we want to cry out, "I want my mommy!"

In the first days after surgery, Glenna was moved out of intensive care into a room of her own. Early in the morning, she was alone and having coughing spasms because of the tracheostomy tube in her throat. She felt she was suffocating, alone. Her friend and business partner Emerson arrived—with a teddy bear and child's magic slate to use for writing. Glenna wrote him a note: "Stay with me and hold my hand, don't leave me until Curtis gets here, I'm afraid." She was like a fearful child who needed an adult to provide safety and comfort.

There is also a humiliating aspect to regression, when it feels yucky and self-defeating. Sometimes, when I am really upset and out of control, I feel utterly dependent on others. I completely forget that I am a competent, independent adult; on any other day, I could prove that to you in a second. Instead, I demand help and attention from others and, if I don't get it *right away,* have been known to whine and snivel and then end up hating myself and feeling ashamed about my clinging.

One embarrassing example of regression occurred while Glenna and I were working on this book. As often happened, my anxieties were stirred up by delving back into our cancer experiences. We had developed a work schedule for the weekend, because we had much to accomplish and our time together was limited. Then Glenna was interrupted by a series of telephone calls that I thought she should not have taken. After all, we were supposed to be working together, but if she kept talking on the phone, then I couldn't write anything more and then I'd have to go home with nothing done and then the book would never get finished—the imagined failures and my help-lessness escalated. The longer Glenna talked on the phone, the higher my anxiety got, the greater my need for her attention and my anger for not getting it. It never occurred to me to go on to one of the many tasks that didn't require interaction. I was anxious and dependent on Glenna to take care of me.

We talked about what was happening and were able to label my behavior and understand what had triggered it and why. The insight I got from this naming was enormously helpful to me afterward in feeling more control over my responses to fear. When we are able to put a name to what we are doing and can understand why we need to do it (because we are deeply afraid and feel helpless, as we may have as children), we can stop being so hard on ourselves.

Learning to Live with Fear

As I write, I look back to the time I entered limbo, and I see how far I have come in a short period of time. Then, I had no idea I was even *in* limbo. I had no way to understand and orga-nize the jumble of fears and defenses that were rattling around inside me. With distance, I see that over time I learned there was a rhythm to my cycle of fear, hope, and comfort.

After five years of living with his own cycles postcancer, Brian saw that the reappearance of both fear and optimism was predictable.

> I am, in fact, still very paranoid about my cancer coming back. The paranoia is not a general, background sort of thing. Instead, I am absolutely confident of survival on about twenty-seven days of any month, and I am reasonably sure that I am going to die on the other three days (usually on three days in succession). My wife, Dianne, even gets to play along. The other day I had a red, inflamed eye that felt very much as though I had scratched it or had something in it. Dianne said, "Can you get melanoma of the eye?" I, of course, said yes. Life goes on.

We learn our own rhythms through a combination of self-reflection and feedback from others. I learned which friends could tolerate me when I was feeling out of control and using regressive behavior. Sometimes they were friends who had also had cancer. Their acceptance of me helped me to accept myself and trust that there was a good reason for the way I was feeling. I wasn't just being crazy, even though I felt that way.

Identifying Triggering Events

A major step in learning to live with fear is to identify what can trigger our fears. Some common triggers have already been mentioned: a doctor's appointment, an anniversary of diagnosis or surgery, the death of someone close. In addition, there may be triggers that are unique to our experience. For me, many acts associated with this book activated my fear: interviewing survivors, reading my old journals, discussing the concepts, writing about cancer.

When we can identify our triggers, we set a powerful and freeing process in motion. We can begin the identification with silent questions: What is going on here? Why do I feel out of control? Why am I behaving this way? What am I anxious about? We may be able to trace our feelings back to a chance remark or a stray thought or event that set our anxiety off and running.

Once we have labeled the trigger, we are able to see our reaction as logical and normal. And we can then link our behavior to the reason for it. Once we understand this predictable chain of responses, we can admire the coherence and creativity of our mind-body system and the way in which we are trying to protect ourselves.

Earlier in this chapter, Katharine developed some physical symptoms that frightened her. The deaths of two childhood friends triggered her anxiety because she was reminded that she, too, was vulnerable to death and unable to control fate. Her stomach then distended with gas, a physical response that mirrored her fear that she had developed tumors in her abdomen.

Martina is an attorney and mediator in her forties who was successfully treated for non-Hodgkin's lymphoma eight years before her interview. She gained insight from her cancer: she discovered that whenever she begins to worry about a recurrence, it is a signal that she is neglecting her need for creative expression.

> There are times that I get off track for quite a while and don't make art, and I know that that's the thing that satisfies my soul that I need to do. . . . I've had periods when I worry. . . . And when I find myself worrying, it's hooked into knowing that I'm not living my life the way I want to be living it. So I feel this tremendous anxiety when I'm stressed day in and day out for any length of time and not happy with what I'm doing. And I recognize that that's when I'm sort of feeling around for lumps and I go, "Oh, I see what's happening."

Accepting Help from Others

Our partners or close friends may recognize our weird behavior even before we do. Through their observations, we can make an educated deduction about what is going on and take steps to soothe our anxiety. It is often a great gift to ourselves and to the people closest to us to include them in this process. Even if they are not skilled at identifying what is going on with us, the simple act of sharing our feelings can be a relief to all concerned.

But it is also true that because they love us, some people may not be able to tolerate discussions that touch upon death anxiety. We have to be sensitive to others' responses to this material, and we have to understand that for some among our friends and family, these discussions will be off limits.

For these reasons, a social worker, counselor, or therapist may be the most appropriate person for us to talk with first, particularly when we have just ended treatment and are learning to live with the heightened awareness of our mortality. He or she will have the skills to help us sort through the issues and make sense of them, so we can begin to share them with our friends and family coherently.

Glenna and I both chose to work with psychotherapists. Glenna went into traditional analysis after her cancer. I was already in therapy with a psychologist when I became ill. Glenna has written about the importance of this relationship to her in Chapter Two. For me, knowing I had a regular time to talk with Steve, my therapist, about cancer, life, and death made me feel more secure. His steady reliability in the face of my pain, and his ability to help me understand the many layers of thoughts and feelings related to my relationships made our sessions together often feel like being taken aboard a life raft.

Some people are not comfortable with the idea of talking with a professional. Even when they do want to talk, finding the right counselor can feel scary. There are books available to help you find, interview, and select an appropriate professional helper. The most important criterion is that you feel comfortable with the person, that from the outset, the counselor understands your messages, spoken and unspoken. If you do not have an immediate sense of trust and empathy, interview others until you feel that sense of "rightness."

Learning What Calms Our Fear

As we learn what triggers our fears, we also learn what calms them. Over time, I learned that I got anxious a few days before a regular medical checkup. I also knew that I wouldn't connect my anxiety with the appointment. Instead, I would worry about my work or my lover. Then I would spend futile time trying to fix the wrong thing. I finally asked my friends to remind me why I was anxious at those times, that the anxiety was a perfectly normal reaction. Then I could accept my worrying instead of fighting it. The act of saying to myself, "You're anxious, and it's okay to be anxious now, and it will pass," provided comfort. Sometimes I even felt better.

My fear around checkups really played itself out in my doctor's waiting room. He is notoriously late for appointments, and I would be in a rage by the time I finally got in to see him. Eventually, I told him that waiting like that made my anxiety intolerable and asked if there was something he could please do about it. His staff arranged my future appointments to be the first ones after lunch, before his schedule got behind. They thought it was amusing that I was so upset, but I didn't care. I had recognized my own anxiety and done something active to manage it.

Because Glenna's cancer was at the base of her tongue, the lymph nodes nearby were the focus of her fear. For the first year after her surgery, she felt those nodes at least weekly if not daily, and occasionally, one would be swollen. She developed a ritual for calming her terror. First, she always got somebody else to feel the nodes—either her doctor or her husband. Then she either wrote in her journal her worst fears and fantasies (surgery, radiation, deathbed scenes), to get the fear outside her, or she would call a friend who could understand her terror without escalating it. Finally, she would lie down, put on soothing music, and visualize herself in a peaceful, beautiful place in nature, relaxed and comfortable. Then she would be able to go on with the day. This sequence took time and discipline, but it was how Glenna began to manage the beginning of limbo. Over time, the entire sequence was no longer necessary; she could gain relief by just writing or talking or meditating.

Virginia, the survivor who is a psychologist and trained to pay attention to internal processes, articulates what she does with her fear: "There is fear all the time; you live with it. It's there every single day. Most of the time, you're not aware of it. January, when they thought I'd had a recurrence, brought me into the awareness. I try to do what [author] Steven Levine talks about as 'soft belly'—live with the fear and not tighten around it. Then you're not paralyzed by the fear, but you allow it to be there."

There are many techniques to soothe anxiety that we have all probably used: getting a massage, having a warm bath, taking a walk, going to a movie, exercising, meditating, listening to tapes of the ocean or the wind, watching the behavior of birds. Anything that takes you out of yourself and stops the repetitive cycle of worry is something you can use for this kind of anxiety too.

Seeing the Other Side of Fear

Once we become more comfortable with the new reality that we have very little control over when and how we will die, we can begin to focus our energy on *how* we live now. This can free us from worrying about something that is really out of our hands. It can actually be a comfort to feel we can give up the exhausting and unprofitable pastime of second-guessing fate.

David Spiegel, a psychiatrist at Stanford University, has been working for many years with women whose breast cancer has spread throughout their bodies. In support groups, these women talk about their feelings concerning the probability that they will die from their cancer, and about how they want to live in the time that is left for them. In *Living Beyond Limits,* Spiegel says that the most important lesson for him was that these dying women were able to find satisfaction and even deep joy in their lives in ways they had not before they had cancer.

When we hang on to the illusion that we can control our fate and somehow prevent our own deaths, we invest energy in a useless exercise. The reality is that we will all die, and unless we kill ourselves, we cannot choose the time and circumstances. Given the fact that our remaining time to live is limited (whether it is one year or forty years), it seems ridiculous to use precious energy in denying death and worrying about a future we cannot know. It wears us down and keeps us miserable. If we can do it, we are better off using our need to control in choosing how we spend our time today. As Virginia says, "Almost daily, I'll say, 'This is my last day; how can I be with it more fully?'"

Sometimes just reminding ourselves, "Hey, I don't know what's going to happen. So what can I do today, right now, that is satisfying," can be a relief. It takes the pressure off. It gives us different questions to ask ourselves. Rather than spinning our wheels around things that have no answer—What's going to happen to me? Will my cancer come back? What can I do to keep it from coming back?—our questions become, What will give me satisfaction today? What would I regret if I died tomorrow? These questions help us experience the here and now as well as act on dreams and fantasies for a better life.

Dorothy, the business consultant who is a breast cancer survivor, came to this same conclusion:

> At one point with my cancer, it felt to me like I was on death row, and I was in a cell waiting for my execution. Even though I feel healthy and I'm fine, you always have in the back of your mind that, "hm, I wonder when D day is actually going to pop up here." . . . It's moved into the background some, but I think about cancer every day, about the fact that I've got it, that I've had it. . . . And basically, I just kind of think no one's got a lease on life, and before I go, I'm going to try to live life to the fullest, and if that's forty years from now, that's great, and if it's four years from now, well, then I'm going to say I've had a great forty-six years.

The earthy sense of being alive that I felt in the middle of my death terror is the other side of fear. I began to look for that other side when I was afraid. The first time I remember doing this consciously was in my cancer support group when two members were close to death. Earlier in my recovery, I identified fully with their dying and would leave the group flattened by fear for myself. Later, I was able to tolerate participating in their dying process by deliberately reminding myself that I was alive and healthy now and that life is to be savored.

When our fear first surfaces, it feels intolerable. We try to get rid of it any way we can. It is scary to feel sucked into that dark internal mess the first few times. If we are gentle with ourselves and remember that we are recovering from a trauma and are doing the best we can under very difficult circumstances, our courageous exploration of our fears will eventually bring some order to the chaos. We are taking our first shaky steps in limbo. Slowly, we will begin to dance.

5

Beginning to Dance:
Grieving Our Losses

*I was recovering from surgery and still feeling lucky when my
wise friend Susan dropped by with two small booklets. They were
about grief, written by Protestant ministers for their widowed
parishioners. I thought, "How strangely inappropriate," but
nodded in thanks . . . and put the books aside. I hadn't lost anyone or anything. In fact, I had been given an incredible gift—
my own life. I had nothing to grieve. The surgery had not been
deforming. I still had my face. I had only part of a tongue, so
my speech was badly slurred, but I was determined to learn to
talk again. I reflected on my friend's thoughtfulness—wistfully.
She didn't really understand me.*

*For the next several weeks, speech was beyond me, chewing and
swallowing food took up most of my time. I couldn't concentrate
on any of the books I had planned to read, but I was able to
write in my journal, and mysteriously, I was able to read the
grief pamphlets. They were more interesting than I had
expected, although they had little to do with me.*

*It took me a while to register that I was grieving, but the anxi-
ety and confusion, the feelings of sadness and loss that the ministers described, obviously resonated within me, or the booklets
would never have held my attention. I can now recognize that
I took more comfort from my friend's gift than I knew. She
understood me better than I did.*

GLENNA

:r cancer, I had many losses to grieve. However, in my
horia at the prospect of survival, I was oblivious to my
was just as well, since I was not yet physically or emo-
ᵗᵒⁿᵃˡˡʸ strong enough to face that pain. Even on a good day,
I hate grief because it means that I have lost someone or something I dearly loved and did not want to lose. The pain is nearly
unbearable. In the immediate aftermath of diagnosis and
surgery, I had not had enough good days. I was not prepared
to think about grief, much less feel its pain. Consequently, I
was in mourning before I knew what was going on.

It took six months for me to recognize my grief. It happened when my father-in-law died and I started crying in my
sleep. Distressing sounds would wake me in the night, and in
my confusion, I would slowly realize that those sounds were
me, sobbing out my pain. My feelings about his death were so
entangled with my own memories and fears of cancer that I
realized the knot in my heart and belly and mind was all one
knot: grief. Finally, I could ask myself, "What have *I* lost?"
instead of pushing the idea away.

When we survive cancer, we lose more of ourselves than I
can name. Who we were and what we thought our life would be
is gone. We have had a disease from which we could have died;
at times, we probably thought we would, and we still may. Even
if we live, we will never get our old selves back. We will never
see the world through our old eyes, and we will never be seen
by others as we were seen before. That is more than enough to
account for our grief, but unfortunately, it's not all.

There are also the physical losses and what they mean to us
as well as others. There are tangible losses: money, career, insurance coverage, relationships, plans for the future, and on and
on. And there are intangible losses: a global sense of certainty,
our beliefs about our future, our safety, and our ability to control our lives. As Martina observed in her interview, "*Nothing*
has ever been the same since I had cancer." Nothing is the same,
and everything that has changed must be grieved. Dorothy
summed it up this way: "There's a grieving process that we just

have to go through . . . because we've had something that basically changed our whole life for the rest of our life."

Most of the survivors talked about their losses and their grief. Although many of them concluded that their grief left them sadder but wiser, each experience of grief, and its expression, was unique. This should come as no surprise. We are who we are—individuals—and we bring our unique history of grief to our cancer and our survival.

Our experiences with grief begin very early in life, and as with all things deeply personal and real, those early experiences shape everything that follows. My parents' lives were marked by early and traumatic losses, and they carried throughout their lives the burden of unresolved grief. Some of their grief was passed on to me in the hushed tone of our household. My first memory of grief that I can name is of my father's grief when his father died and its effect on me. Although I was only six, this story reveals much about me now as well as then.

At the end of my nightly bath, I would call for my father. After he had checked behind my ears to see if I had done my job, he would pull the plug and, at my request, turn out the light as he left the room. In the tub, alone and in the dark, I played a secret game. I had to dry myself and climb out before the water swirled down the drain. If I lost the race, my body would be pulled through the plumbing into the ground beneath our house. Alternately, I imagined that snakes, who always live in plumbing fixtures, would slither out and get me. Every night I won my race, and every night I worried about dark holes—about being sucked down or what might slip out.

Like every childhood game, this was serious business. I was coping with something I did not yet understand. I knew that my grandfather had just died. I remember the telegram and my father's swollen eyes. I also know that this was the time my favorite aunt, my father's favorite sister, was dying of cancer. Daddy was my anchor throughout childhood, my safe place. Now he didn't always hear me when I spoke. Sometimes he didn't even see me in the room. "Oh, you're here," he would say. "When did you come in?" I did not know what dying meant. I also could not know that I had regressed—I was much too old to be afraid of disappearing down the drain. But I sensed that somehow life could break your heart.

Now that I have known death in my own body, I also know survival's cruel paradox. Cancer was an open sore, a tiny lump, a small black hole that could swallow me up. Survival has meant facing death, daily, in more small ways than I can count. This time it is not a game that I have made up, and there is no way to escape. For survivors, daily life is filled with fear—of danger lurking in our bodies, of unanticipated losses, and of death.

As adults, we learn to live with fear and loss and death. It is a little like my game in that it is a daily task. Most of us need help to mourn our losses. It is simply too hard and too lonely to grieve alone: we need a witness. Both Lisa and I have needed all the help that we could get—from each other, from family and friends, and from our therapists.

Physical Losses

All cancer survivors have sustained physical damage. We have sacrificed part of our bodies in the hope that we will live. Given our choices, it was worth the sacrifice, but that does not ease the loss. Remember, it was a choice between bad and worse. Among the survivors interviewed for this book, Judy said it most directly: "I had to keep my focus. I wanted to live. That's what made it worth sacrificing my breast." But she didn't minimize the loss: "Living for a year and a half without a breast really got my attention. It gave me time for grieving and adjusting. I felt a lot of pain and sorrow." Then, reflecting on her treatment choices, she observed: "The whole thing is just shit. So you make the best choice you can." That about sums it up.

Many of the survivors interviewed live with disabilities and scars. My scars are inside my mouth, so they are invisible, even to me. Once I had learned to talk again, I tried to put the memories of my disability out of mind, just as my scars are out of sight. In fact, every time I speak, the effort that it takes reminds me that I have had cancer and lived to tell the tale. But I have never before told anyone what it was like to learn to talk again. The base of my tongue on the right side and the adjacent floor of my mouth were cut away. Without that muscle attachment, my tongue sits sideways, and what was once its right side now functions as the tip. That side is partially scar tissue, so it is thickened and stiff. If you twist your tongue crosswise in your mouth and try to talk, you will get a sense and a little of the sound of what my speech was like.

I had to retrain my mouth and lips to make the old sounds with this clumsy tongue as their instrument. The whole process was bizarre, beginning with my denial. Although all the doctors I consulted mentioned their concern for my future speech, I just didn't get it. When my surgeon teased that I might not have "as quick a tongue" when he was finished with me, I heard the words, but some combination of denial and my will to live at almost any cost kept me from their meaning.

For the first week after surgery, I could not speak at all. On day five, when my surgeon pulled the naso-gastric tube out, Curtis and my brother, Ed, were amazed when I tried to speak. I wanted to say thank you to my doctor, and I tried, but when he left my room, Curtis and Ed burst into laughter. They wanted to know where I had found the gall to say "F———— you!" to my surgeon! But that's not what I had said at all.

At first, I just made sounds, and no one understood me. Within a month, I sounded exactly like a fourth-grade boy at the "poverty project" where I had done volunteer work when I was in high school. I can still see that skinny kid with no shoes and what we called a "harelip" (*cleft palate* is the medically and politically correct term). His upper lip and the entire roof of his mouth gaped open, and his words were full of forced air and impossible to understand. Periodically, the other kids would circle him on the playground and mimic his sounds, pointing and laughing until he cried. I had that kid's speech.

Even after several more months of constant practice, I sounded drunk, and I continued to sound that way for months.

That was a wondrous and terrible time. I did most of my work by writing from home. The phone was useless. Not even Curtis could understand me on it. He would call and talk to me, but I could not talk back. Every day, I spent hours making sounds, the way some young children vocalize continuously as they learn to speak. Since I was alone, I talked to myself all the time—a running slurred commentary on everything I did. I read whatever I wrote out loud as I composed. Like a child, I would say, "Now I'm getting up to go to the bathroom." "Now I'm going to make my lunch. Down the stairs, open the refrigerator (that's a hard word), let's see what we have here." I was amazed by my patience with myself and by how fascinating it was to hear this voice of mine. I loved its wacky sound because it still had a sound and that meant that I was still here—alive and carrying on.

However, as the months passed, I got bored with narrating my limited daily life and afraid that I might sound like this forever. My surgeon was encouraging but frank. He and I did not know if my speech would improve further, and I became increasingly aware of other people's reactions to me. My family and closest friends were loyal and patient. Both Curtis and Kyle learned to read my lips. They would look me in the eye, smile encouragingly, and struggle to understand. Several friends tactfully suggested speech therapists who had helped their children, and I dutifully recorded the names. But others who knew me looked away when I spoke. I understood, and I still hated them for it. Strangers frequently behaved as if I did not exist. I remember trying to pay a young cashier at the grocery store. We had had several brief exchanges as she went through my shopping cart, and her tone seemed impatient. When I asked her to repeat the amount I owed, she turned to the woman behind me in the checkout line and said, "Why don't alcoholics stay at home?" If looks could kill, I would have murdered her. I walked away in tears.

Such exchanges were a daily event—at the gas station, the dry cleaners, the bank. Anytime I had to do business with a stranger, I risked being treated with contempt. But it was actually a problem with more than strangers. I suspect that only my capacity for denial allowed me to go on. Months later, a colleague told me that throughout our first conversation after my surgery, which he had known nothing about, he assumed that I had become addicted to Valium. I was mortified. He reminded me that he had been in medical practice long enough to know the symptoms—and that good people could become addicted. Images of Betty Ford on national television graciously acknowledging Gerald Ford's defeat with slurred speech flashed through me.

I was also filled with fleeting memories and sensations from very early childhood when I had learned to talk the first time. There is an entry in my baby book, in my mother's careful hand. The book asks parents to fill in the "Number of words in child's vocabulary." In the blank, my mother wrote, "?? Glenna was never at a loss for words after 22 months." But I can now remember being at a loss. I would know the word I wanted to form, but my "tang got tungled" (one of my expressions from childhood), and the word would come out wrong. I would try and try until I wanted to explode. At thirty-seven, that feeling was nearly as old as I was, and I was feeling it again.

I persevered. It took an entire year before I could talk respectably. Ten years later, my speech is different than it was before my surgery, slower and more deliberate, but that is something most other people never notice. When I am very tired or very cold, my speech is still noticeably impaired.

As I recall my year of relearning, I hear the words of two other survivors. Judy said: "While you're in it, you don't realize how awful it really is. You're just getting through it. Then you look back and realize: that was just awful." It was. And along with Socorro, I feel like a very "lucky" lady. That is a painful truth of survival: luck and loss are intertwined.

The specific issues of physical disability and rehabilitation are beyond the scope of this book. What I want to convey here is that to be physically impaired or disfigured may create functional problems or feelings that are so oppressive as to crowd out other considerations for a time. If you have sacrificed a vital portion of your body in the hope that you will live, I not only respect the magnitude of your loss, I also recognize that highly visible physical losses change not only our self-images but also the way others treat us in innumerable subtle and not-so-subtle ways. A major physical change is a constant reminder that we are someone new.

Comparing Our Losses

We cancer patients do a curious thing when we compare our losses to those of others. Research by Shelley Taylor has revealed that we usually compare ourselves with someone who has in our estimation suffered a greater loss. We feel pity for that other patient, and we count our own blessings. We know that we are fortunate, by contrast. Thus the woman with a simple mastectomy might compare herself to another who has had a recurrence in her other breast but not with the woman whose lumpectomy proved successful. We want to feel better about our own fate, not worse, and we choose our comparisons accordingly.

The Meaning of Our Losses

What matters even more than the physical loss is the highly personal meaning of what has been lost. This was true for Lisa and me and was borne out by research by Michael Speca and his colleagues. We each attach a different significance to different parts of our bodily self. One person's defacing scar is another's badge of courage. Three of the breast cancer survivors interviewed had breast reconstruction and were very happy with the results, while for other women, part of the enduring meaning of the event was embodied in what was now missing.

For logistical reasons, Judy chose to have her reconstruction a year and a half after her mastectomy, but looking back, she saw that period of experiencing what she had lost as facilitating her grief. In contrast, both Barbara and Charlotte had immediate reconstruction and were confident that they had made the right choice for them.

For my mother, who refused even to wear a prosthesis, life without her breast was part of her larger commitment to realism. It was an unspoken way of saying, "This is my life. I am a woman who has survived cancer. If it shows, it shows."

We also attach our own meaning to being healthy, to seeing ourselves as healthy people. Bente has been physically sick for much of her life. From an early age, she had to live within the limitations of a serious lung disease. As a child, she found ways to enjoy life and feel good about herself even though she was not like other children. In contrast to Bente's experience, I have always thought of myself as extremely healthy—those were the words I always checked on medical history forms. Consequently, having a life-threatening illness, incapacitating surgery, and a long recovery period during which I could not talk was more than a physical ordeal, it was an emotional trial.

With the diagnosis of cancer, my sense of self was on the line. After cancer, I was not robust and healthy; I was frail, and I knew that I could die. I am normally slim, and with the stress of surgery, I had lost ten pounds of muscle mass. I remember glimpsing my naked body in the mirror as I stepped from my bath. I not only looked like an anorexic, in profile I was so thin that I had the fleeting image of my body disappearing. It was unnerving. In truth, my former sense of self had disappeared. Before cancer, I had seen the world as conveniently divided— the healthy and the sick, the living and the dying. Now the lines were blurred.

Practical Losses

Beyond the physical losses and their implications, other losses are waiting to be tallied. What is the effect of our cancer and its treatment on our important relationships? On partner? Children? Parents? Friends? If someone important has let us down, we may be grieving that disappointment. If our children are frightened and sad, we ache for them as well. Brian's feelings about his family go to the heart of survivor grief: "My overriding feeling, especially during the first few months, was a deep and desperate sense of failure. I was in a forlorn depression over my possible inability to do the one thing that I wanted most— to safely raise my children to be good and happy adults. That would be my personal tragedy, beyond everything else."

What is the impact of our cancer on our careers? Plans? Salaries? Insurance? On our favorite pastimes? The list goes on, depending on your cancer and your life-style. In this way, surviving cancer is a lot like having your home burglarized. You find more things missing as time goes by, and each time you find something else, even if it is something small, you feel robbed all over again.

Intangible Losses

We have not finished counting our losses. The deepest ones are intangible. We have lost our most basic assumptions about ourselves and the world. We assumed that we had a future; now we don't know. We assumed that we were safe in our own bodies; now we can't be sure. We assumed that we had more control over our own lives. If we did the right things, we would be all right. In general, we believed in a more certain world.

Many of us began to lose our sense of certainty with the difficult treatment decisions that we faced. No matter what we did or did not do, there were no guarantees. Some of us had to make harder choices than others. There is no arguing that it is easier to have a mole removed than our bowels even though, when all is said and done, the melanoma survivor may face the same or greater risk of recurrence as the colon cancer survivor. As we make treatment decisions based on our risk of future death, we realize that the numbers do not tell us anything about our individual chances of survival. Brian understood this all too well: "The debriefing at the Melanoma Center was generally depressing, but the news that other men with similar malignant moles on their backs had a mortality rate of only about 20 percent was heartening. As a scientist, however, I understood that statistics are only useful for making predictions about large groups of people. I knew that I was either going to be all the way alive or all the way dead. So the statistics were not as comforting as I might have hoped."

I, too, longed for comforting assurances that I was not to get. Surgery was my best treatment option, and all the specialists I consulted were unanimous—my surgeon was the best. Then my internist called. He had heard through the hospital grapevine about my cancer and wanted to give me some advice. He was characteristically direct: "They want to do surgery. Have they leveled with you on your survival odds? You know, it may not be worth it, and you need to find out for yourself. How much of your speech will you lose? Have they told you about that?" I could not answer his questions, and that is how I came to spend that dreadful day in the medical school library finding the answers for myself.

It was hard to judge survival odds because the number of reported cases of tumors detected as early as mine was so small—twenty, to be exact. There was nothing in the literature of the time about speech after surgery. So I moved into the unknown, literate on the subject but not well informed. The information did not exist. After I had recovered from surgery, my brother and sister-in-law gave me an apron imprinted with the motto "Life is uncertain. Eat dessert first." It was the perfect, painful, private joke.

The Loss of Cherished Illusions

We may be slow to reckon the intangible damage. The loss of cherished illusions is hard to admit. We tell ourselves that we always knew that we would die—someday. Nothing has really changed. We had not believed in our own invulnerability since adolescence—we claim. In fact, we may lose some pride in making the admission that we all believed that nothing bad could happen to us, despite the evidence. And we all believed in our heart of hearts that we would not die. As Lisa said, she believed there was an order to the universe and she had a secure place in it. That none of us has absolute security anywhere, and certainly not in anything as large as the universe, is intolerable. So we all proceed "as if."

The Loss of Our Certain Future

Brian was acutely aware that he had lost his faith in the future: "I could no longer count on a long, leisurely life. I lost all interest in long-term personal or professional planning, and I could not get excited about things that might have a long-term payout. . . . I generally became a self-centered victim in a play with an unknown number of acts."

Similarly, there was a period after her metastasis when Lisa's reply to almost everything was, "I don't have enough time." She finally heard what she was saying: "I was expressing my subliminal awareness that my lifetime was finite."

Charlotte also worries about the future: "I can't stand the thought of the children— . . . I would be devastated if I knew that they wouldn't have me anymore." When she and her husband have conversations about what they will do when the children are grown, she says, "Most of the time, I think, 'Well, you can do it. I probably won't be there.'"

Ellen carries her worries about a future to their painful conclusion: "When you live as a cancer survivor, you don't know what your future is going to be. . . . I'm not able to put words to some of the powerful exploration I've done around death, or around facing the fears. . . . I think I'm still dealing with death. I've not come to peace around that." It is slim consolation to know that few of us come to peace around the loss of our own future.

The Loss of Our Sense of Safety

Jeannette was in her late seventies when she spoke with us and already dealing with issues of aging and mortality. But having cancer felt different. It was "this other kind of feeling, that you never know what's going to strike. . . . I'm not sure why there is such an insidious quality to cancer. With a heart condition, it's not something that's invading your body, but with cancer, people think that there's *something* in there."

Many of us feel a sense of alienation from our own bodies after cancer, as if our bodies have disappointed us in some essential way. And they may do it again. When Ellen discovered a lump in her breast one year after her melanoma, she had it checked. The biopsy revealed a condition that put her at greater risk for breast cancer. Ellen said, "When that happened, I wondered if my body was just this bad cell producer. It was really terrifying." Feeling that we are not safe in our own bodies is terrifying. That is when Ellen found a psychotherapist who had experience with cancer patients. In her therapy, Ellen realized, "I'd done a number on myself . . . I was damaged goods." As she continued to grieve her "damage," she came to a crucial awareness, "I had really changed, and I had kept thinking that I would go back to exactly who I was before having the melanoma." Then she was able to grieve the loss of her old self.

The Loss of Illusions of Control

When Barbara's breast cancer recurred, the obvious futility of her efforts to control her fate was central to her pain: "Tears were just streaming down my face. All of a sudden, I thought: 'I've really been a good kid. I've watched the fats I take into my diet; I've exercised; I barely have caffeine. I lead a really healthy life. What's going on?'" Barbara's sense that she had been "a good kid" is exactly to the point. At a deep and often unconscious level, we believe what we were taught as children: if we are good enough, things will turn out fine. Letting go of that cherished illusion is painful.

Neil argued that "with cancer, you need to come to an acceptance of your fragility—that you're vulnerable and that you will die. [To deny that reality] panders to the pathology of the omnipotent child, to that illusion of control." Neil believes that

e as a cancer survivor "is very much like the serenity prayer
lcoholics Anonymous]: I acknowledge the limits of my
control."

I had a poignant experience several years after my cancer. A
colleague invited me to lunch. We had always respected each
other's work, and I especially enjoyed her keen intelligence and
the precision of her thinking. Over lunch, she told me that she
had a confession to make. My cancer had terrified her—for herself as well as for me. She had believed, without ever knowing it,
that she was safe from such diseases. When I got cancer, she knew
for the first time that anyone could, and that meant that she was
not safe. My cancer had robbed her of a basic assumption. I knew
exactly what she had lost. I had lost the same illusion.

Mourning It All

As it turns out, all of our losses must be grieved, visible and
invisible, large and seemingly small. It is the highly personal
meaning of what has been lost that determines our grief, not
the loss per se. We facilitate the grief process by honoring what
we have lost, not minimizing it. Contrary to popular wisdom,
counting your blessings and keeping a stiff upper lip is bad
advice.

While we are in the depths of this special sadness, it is reassuring to know that grief is a process and that it is already in
motion. We won't feel this awfulness forever, but we also cannot rush through it. Since the purpose of grief is to integrate a
new, and unwanted, reality, it proceeds by fits and starts. We
reject the new reality, but it won't go away. Our identity is
changed. We cannot go back to who we were before. We have
already tried that, and it didn't work. We let in a little more
awareness of our losses, then shut down again. We feel the loss
more keenly, then back off again. And again and again. Gradually, we can hold the losses in our mind without feeling that
we will be destroyed.

A Short Course on Grief

After we wake up in limbo, we are disoriented and confused. Our moods vary from a sense of letdown to genuine depression. We are distracted, filled with memories of diagnosis and treatment that aren't like memories at all they are so immediate and vivid. We may see images from diagnosis and treatment, hear snatches of dialogue. It is almost as if we carry a movie inside us, the picture and the sound are out of sync, and fragments from the reel play, uninvited, in our heads. While the film is rolling, there is always something more we should be doing, but who has the time or energy? We are irritable, sometimes angry at the world or the people we love most. Why can't they understand? And things keep going wrong, or if they don't, we know they could. We cannot stop wondering, What if? Everywhere we turn, we see that something bad could happen.

This is grief, and it is running parallel to our daily life. When we are grieving, we feel beside life, not really in it. We eat but do not taste the food; we sleep but not well. We go through the motions of love and work and play, but we are barely there. Even worse than feeling half-dead are the silent secret moments when we think we are going crazy. In grief, feeling crazy is the norm.

Much is known about the usual grief process. Useful books on this topic have been written by John Bowlby, Richard Kalish, Colin Parkes, and Beverly Raphael (these are listed in the chapter references). It may be helpful to look at the natural course of thoughts and feelings that are characteristic of grief. The similarities between the tasks of grief and the challenges of learning to dance in limbo are striking.

In both grief and limbo, initially we feel numb. There is a blunting of feelings and a sense of disbelief. The loss simply is not real, cannot be real. Nearly all of the cancer survivors interviewed experienced this numb sense of unreality at the time of diagnosis.

People who are grieving a death go on to experience a combination of anger, agitation, anxiety, restlessness, and physical complaints. They search for who and what they have lost, and in their searching, they seem preoccupied and forgetful. That was what was happening in my childhood when my grandfather died and my father did not seem to see or hear me. He was lost in thoughts and feelings about his own father and memories of their relationship. Often the bereaved are reviewing the relationship or replaying events associated with the death. They experience a painful yearning for what has been lost. These symptoms of grief resemble cancer survivors' mix of thoughts and feelings as we struggle to understand Why me? and experience the confusion of waking up in limbo.

The bereaved also experience disorganization, anger, depression, and despair as the reality of their loss sinks in. That's how many of us feel when we are fully awake in limbo. Interestingly, in the grief process there is a temptation to mitigate the loss through denial or illusions. The bereaved may refuse to talk about the death or may speak of the dead person as if she or he is still alive. They may set a place at the table for the person or carry on a conversation with him or her. We face similar temptations. Many cancer survivors vow to carry on as if nothing has happened. Some will not speak of their cancer. Others redouble efforts to control their fate through rigid diets, "magical" pills, or devotion to a "savior."

Gradually, those who grieve are able to relinquish the past. Their sadness over the loss of what is no more becomes bearable. The loss is real but not ever present. I remember knowing that I was truly on the mend when I got bored with my cancer experience. Finally, I was ready for something more than my preoccupation with myself and my survival. I needed more in my life, and I could actually concentrate on something other than my tongue. For a while, my entire universe had been the lower right quadrant of my face. Nothing else existed, much less mattered.

Ultimately, the bereaved reorganize themselves and their lives around the new reality. A similar redefinition of ourselves is the goal of those of us who would dance in limbo. In grief and in survival, our ultimate task is to make sense of our new reality.

How Survivor Grief Is Different

Survivor grief is different from bereavement in two important ways. First, it has a different and often less apparent cause. In bereavement, we know what we are grieving. The most commonly recognized grief occurs when someone important to us has died, or we are facing our own impending death. For cancer survivors, the biggest losses are intangible and the paradox of grieving our good fortune is almost too much to bear. At moments, it is difficult to remember that we are not grieving only the possibility of our untimely death, we are grieving the deep knowledge of our eventual death and all the other losses catalogued here.

For cancer survivors, survivor grief also has a different and more confusing course. In bereavement, there is no high. Cancer survivors' grief begins, like any other grief, with disbelief and shock. When the shock wears off, we feel blind fear. That sensation of numb terror is similar to the first pangs of other kinds of grief, but when blind fear becomes blind hope, survivor grief no longer feels like grief at all. We feel powerful and confident, and that is not how grief feels. The fact that most of us do not grieve during treatment throws us off. The process is not only interrupted, but the intervening feelings are so alien to grief that most of us do not recognize our grief when it resumes at treatment's end.

Survivor Grief Is a Delayed Grief

Those who study grief, recognize the phenomenon of delayed grief. A delay typically occurs when survival issues are so compelling that we cannot experience the feelings of grief at the time of the loss. That is exactly what happens to us as cancer patients. Survival issues take all our time and energy until treatment is complete. We cannot afford the luxury of grief until later. Our delayed grief may be triggered by a later loss, such as the death of a pet or illness of a friend. Psychologists now understand that this occurs through the mechanism of displacement. My reaction to my father-in-law's death six months after my cancer surgery was a clear example of delayed grief. His death prompted my first real awareness that I had lost my illusion of immortality. I knew that it could be me in that coffin, and that was an awful thing to know. The interviews Lisa and I had with cancer survivors are replete with examples of delayed grief.

Charlotte felt strong and completely able to cope throughout her own diagnosis and treatment, but when a friend's daughter was diagnosed with leukemia, her own grief found expression: "She was diagnosed one year from the day I was diagnosed with cancer. When I found out, I just kept crying; I couldn't stop." I suspect Charlotte's reaction was much like my own. She mourned for her friend and the daughter, but the added force of the feeling was her own delayed grief.

Socorro also had a delayed grief reaction. She battled breast tumors for five years, beginning with benign tumors that caused bleeding from her nipple and ending with malignant tumors and a mastectomy. Throughout this entire ordeal, which required constant vigilance and three surgeries in four years, she remembers being clear and decisive, "one of those people who wants to bounce back." Remember that Socorro not only bounced back, she continued to see herself as "a very lucky lady." It was four years later, when she had brain surgery for a congenital vascular problem, that she could not "get back to normal." She sought psychotherapy, admitting, "I was a science major, and I'm [good with] facts. Emotions are something I don't deal with very well." Her fear and grief following the brain surgery contained the feelings about breast cancer that she had "laughed off" at the time. She said, "I thought having one breast was pretty funny, but I don't remember laughing a lot after brain surgery." For most of us, having our lives threatened isn't very funny.

Grieving in Limbo

Lisa and I suspect that most of us fail to recognize our grief for a very simple reason. When we wake up in limbo, we do not know what is going on. We had thought we were on top of things. Now we realize we have been largely out of touch with the very real danger to our lives and our deepest feelings about that threat. Our grief is mingled in with our fears of recurrence and all the other confusing feelings. Although we have been feeling lucky, in fact we have ample cause for mourning.

When we wake up in limbo, our grief catches up with us. We will struggle with grief issues repeatedly in the months and years to come, as we slowly work our way toward a resolution. Speed is not our object. Francis Bacon observed that "nature is a labyrinth in which the very haste you move with will make you lose your way." The same is true of grief, which has its own clock and takes its own time. The general rule is that grief takes about two years to run its natural course, and if we try to short-cut the process, we only slow it down.

Lisa and I are at very different stages in the grieving process. During the past six months, Lisa has slowly come to understand that she is in the midst of a powerful grief. She has moved away from the sharp anxieties and fears of recurrence that dominated her inner life for more than a year after her surgery. The theme of fear has been replaced by the theme of loss:

> Only recently have I been able to put words to my experience. I've been walking around for weeks with tears in my throat, ready to spill out unexpectedly. I felt as if layer upon layer of loss and sadness were all bubbling up at once. Everywhere I looked there was a loss. I think this was set off by a time in my love relationship when we were talking about leaving each other. My feelings about losing the man and the relationship overpowered me. I could not separate them from my experiences as a very young child, feeling abandoned and alone, nor from my anger and grief over a burglary at my home in which

several family heirlooms I loved were stolen. Everything was mixed together to create a pervasive darkness inside me. My humor, my optimism, plans for the future, and all sense of hope were missing. I think that as I've begun to mourn the losses associated with my cancer, all the very old losses in my life have been stirred up again and are clamoring to be understood. In a way, I think my cancer has given me the strength to confront and explore the losses I've had in my life. Maybe, by doing this, I can diminish some of the hidden power that years of unexpressed grief have held over me.

Life Is Full of Unacknowledged Losses

We may take a little comfort in the fact that even desired changes entail loss. If we stop to think about it, most of us have been caught off guard by such losses in the past. If we married, we had to give up our single life; if we chose to have a family, we have made many personal sacrifices. Anytime we attain a goal, we achieve the reality, and we lose the dream of it. We hope that it is a good trade, but the losses are nonetheless real. I learned this in my early twenties when some friends had their first child. After years of trying and many disappointments, Suzan was finally pregnant. She and her husband, John, relished the pregnancy. John took beautiful photos of her swollen belly, and they gave the baby in that belly a witty and outrageous name. With the birth, they were elated . . . and unexpectedly sad. I still remember Suzan's painful confession: she had lost the imaginary baby. As she was rejoicing in her beautiful newborn daughter, she was simultaneously grieving the loss of the baby of her dreams.

My own experience is nearly the flip side of the same coin. I had always blindly assumed that I would have children someday. Then, at twenty-six, I fell in love with a divorced man who already had three children. He was committed to them, and he did not want more. My decision to be a stepmother to Curtis's children in place of having my own was agonizing. I suspect that the only reason I was able to choose Curtis instead of children was that I did adore his kids. But my joy in falling in love with someone I thought I could grow old with contained a sacrifice, and I have had to grieve the loss several times. In fact, with menopause, I grieve again. I feel sad, even though I do not regret my decision.

If You Have Survived Other Traumatic Losses

If you have survived other traumatic losses, it is particularly important to grieve the losses from cancer, and it may prove more difficult. As social scientists, both Lisa and I knew that previous experience with trauma is of little use when misfortune strikes again. In part, this is because each trauma is unique, but more to the point, previous traumas are known to leave survivors more, not less, vulnerable. Lisa and I wish this were not so, and despite our knowledge, we each thought, "Damn! I've had experience; I should be better at this." Alas, we were not.

Unfortunately, the belief that what does not kill one makes one stronger is wishful thinking. Each trauma carries its own pain and calls forth the pain of previous trauma. It is important to understand that if you are already a survivor of other traumatic events, the cancer experience may be more difficult for you than for someone whose life has held fewer traumas.

Although I seldom talk about it, I was raped by a neighbor when I was ten. One morning near the end of summer, the "harmless" old man at the end of my block called to me as I skipped past his house. He invited me in for candy—marshmallows, which I have never, ever liked. But I had been taught to respect my elders, so I dutifully walked in. The experience shook me to the core. I suspect that only my father's gentle presence in my daily life and my abiding sense of safety with him saved me from despair. However, that early trauma leaves me especially vulnerable to certain fears—especially to fears of men with sharp objects probing in my body. Fortunately, my surgeon was a wise and gentle man, almost paternal in his protective feelings toward me. It was a perfect fit. But I am wary and still skittish with large men. For all of us who have experienced other traumas and losses, reflecting on the special meaning those painful events lend to the ways we experience our cancer is essential to our well-being, and we may benefit from professional help from a qualified counselor or therapist as we sort out these meanings.

Sadder Is Wiser and Stronger

When we feel sorry for ourselves yet unable to mourn our own losses, we can get mired in self-pity. As I have discussed, self-pity is not a problem, but being mired is. Until we grieve our losses, we can neither respect ourselves as we are now, nor respect the losses of others. It is trite but true: respect and compassion begin with oneself. We cannot give to others what we cannot give ourselves.

Living with a disability has changed me in a way that I am reluctant to confess—my former feelings were so politically and humanely incorrect. It had always been difficult for me to look at severely handicapped people. Their disadvantage made me squirm. I couldn't even carry the thought forward: there but for fortune go I. I simply looked away, not wanting my horror and pity to show. Then I experienced my own disability. In the midst of that first year after surgery, when I still sounded like a drunk, people who knew me took me seriously, and I was able to resume my consulting business. On a flight to a work assignment, my plane made an intermediate stop and a slender middle-aged man with leg braces and crutches boarded. He made his way down the narrow aisle unassisted. I watched, not in horror but in awe. As he passed my seat, our eyes met. I smiled, and I know there was not a trace of pity in my expression because he smiled back. Slowly, and the hard way, I was becoming more whole and human.

It takes tremendous strength and courage to experience sorrow and grief. These powerful emotions are central to human dignity, but that is not what most of us were taught. I like to remember the Classical master in *Alice in Wonderland,* the one who taught Laughing and Grief. It's a brilliant pun, and in real life those skills are far more useful than Latin and Greek. Laughing and grief are natural human reactions to joy and loss, but many of us have to learn how to grieve.

Ellen's experience with melanoma illustrates the necessity of grieving our losses in order to establish our new and positive identities as survivors. Twelve years ago, cancer forced her to think long and hard about her life. She struggled with the meaning of death and with her fears and losses. She hid her scarred leg under kneesocks, and gave up the joy of playing on the beach in the sun. Then she had a breakthrough: "Life became so much easier when I realized that I'm a cancer survivor and this scar is my mark of survival. I became proud of it. The kneesocks disappeared, . . . and when people saw the chunk in my leg . . . I proudly announced, 'I'm a melanoma survivor.'" The scar became an integral part of Ellen's new identity.

Ultimately, our task of survival is to go on about our lives in the full knowledge that we are scarred, visibly and invisibly. We are mortal, and we do not control our fate. And with it all, we are infinitely grateful to be alive. The capacity to grieve our losses is essential to our recovery and to our humanity. Although that grief feels like hell, it is the heart of limbo and the beginning of our dance.

6

Sidestepping the Dance: The Illusion of Control

*When my cancer recurred, my friends desperately wanted to do
something to make me better. They gave me books about positive
thinking, tapes to help me visualize, names of people with strin-
gent miracle diets, recommendations of workshops that would
help me heal by changing my attitudes. I considered all of these
promised remedies, tried the tapes, called for information about
the workshops, read various chapters in the books—and threw up
my hands. "Look," I said to an imaginary audience, "I can't do
this! All these experts are asking me to change my personality,
become a blissed out, stress-free, open and loving vegetarian. If
I could do that, I would have done it by now. There's no way I'm
going to change under this kind of pressure. If the only way
I'm going to beat my cancer is to become someone I am not,
then I say to hell with it."*

LISA

Over and over, I read and was told that I must be positive,
stay calm, not worry. I have always been a worrier, and I
usually study the clouds long before I check for a silver lining.
The more I heard about the necessity for positive thinking in
the face of my cancer, the more terrified I became that because
of who I am, I was going to die. My final decision was to take

103

care of my body and soul as best I could, but the many prescriptions offered to me were appealing. Especially at first, when living with uncertainty was brand new to me. Ultimately, some prescriptions seemed simplistic and gimmicky, and many went against my grain. Nevertheless, the day after I learned my cancer had returned, I bought a juicer that came with anticancer recipes. For weeks, I drank carrot juice twice a day, even though I hated it, and I felt better for doing something, anything. Taking some kind of action relieved my anxiety. I have always known I should eat more vegetables, and hey, this might just be the one antidote to cancer my body had lacked.

Following diets, meditating, and visualizing are all part of the overall rallying of our resources during treatment. All of the survivors interviewed tried out at least one practice that promised to help or cure. And most of us integrated many new practices into our daily routines because they gave us more energy, reduced stress, or generally made us feel better. There is no question that some of these practices are useful and health promoting. It is when we use them to control what is not controllable that we engage in self-delusion. Therefore, we need to look at the expectations we have of any cancer prevention resource that we use.

The Craving for Certainty

As I think back to the time of my diagnosis and treatment, I am surprised that I rejected anything that promised to shrink tumors or banish cancer cells. I was in such a state of shock and fear that my need to believe that I had control over my cancer was enormous. It was a way of avoiding the simple truth that life is uncertain and there are no guarantees.

Many cancer prevention or cure techniques are promoted by their authors as fail-safe, and that promise is the problem. They guarantee outcomes that are simply not possible and hence appeal to our need for a black-and-white world, where there are clear answers to every question. Medical science has not yet discovered the cause of most cancers, nor has it found many reliable cures. No one wants to hear that. Most of us were put in the position of making decisions about treatment for our cancer that we felt unprepared to make. Every decision included trade-offs. When we got the diagnosis, we assumed that our physicians knew what to do about it. When they offered us options and asked us to decide, we were terrified that we would make the wrong treatment choice.

That was our first clue that life with, and after, cancer is uncertain, our first lesson that there are no infallible authorities on life, no absolutes, no clear right or wrong. I hear my therapist's statement to me now: "You are the only authority on your life." Sometimes this thought gives me a feeling of heady power. Sometimes it makes me wail for my mother.

Positive thinking, diets, visualization, and exercise are techniques that reduce stress and anxiety and can help us cope with the side effects of treatment and its aftermath. Whether they give us the edge we need to defeat cancer is unknown. The message of many self-help cancer books, tapes, and workshops, however, is that if you practice what they advocate, you will be safe from recurrence. We may eagerly buy into their promises because we cannot bear to accept that we are in limbo, that no matter what we do we could still get sick, and that no matter how healthy we are now and continue to be, we are still going to die someday.

If we follow certain health-promoting techniques, not to feel better in general but to control matters of life and death, we are sidestepping reality. We are refusing to acknowledge we are in limbo, refusing to learn the steps that are necessary to move gracefully in that land of uncertainty.

A desire for certainty is not restricted to any particular phase in our journey through limbo. It emerges whenever our tolerance for anxiety and painful thoughts is low. For Glenna and me and most of the cancer survivors interviewed for this book, belief in our ability to control fate was strongest during the initial high, when our defense mechanisms were working overtime. During the low, depressing phase, when we first woke up, disoriented, in limbo, some of us continued to cling to the techniques we adopted. The need to know our fate one way or another then reemerged during the painful times when we feared a recurrence of cancer or when we had no answers to the unanswerable questions that crowded us.

Illusions of Control

There is another problem with promises of cure. The message of control they imply cuts both ways. If you have the power to cure your cancer, perhaps you also had the ability to create it. I believe it was this silent message of blame that gave me the most discomfort.

There is a widely held assumption in this country that people with cancer are, in some mysterious way, to blame for their disease. Although the books and tapes that I was given did not say I had created my cancer, the exclusive emphasis on self-help and positive thinking often implied it. Arlene Houlden and other researchers at the University of Pennsylvania recently studied the reasons 234 women who had been diagnosed with breast cancer gave for their cancer. Nearly 40 percent blamed themselves in some way—too much stress in their lives, not getting regular mammograms, negative thinking, being childless, drinking too much coffee, eating too much fat. If this group of women is representative of all women with breast cancer—and the researchers believe it is—that means that 73,000 of the 182,000 U.S. women diagnosed with breast cancer each year feel some degree of guilt about their illness.

This self-blame exists in spite of the fact that these researchers say medical experts "don't have a clue" what causes the vast majority of breast cancers. One of the researchers for this study believes that the current widespread belief in the power of mental attitude plays into this guilt. In some people's minds, the logic becomes black and white: if positive thinking can cure your problems, negative thinking must have created them. Rather than giving us relief, such illusions of control can also make us angry, guilty, and anxious if we cannot do it (whatever "it" is) right, thereby completely defeating the original calming purpose of the positive thinking techniques.

My experience was echoed by many of the cancer survivors to whom Glenna and I spoke. Our friends and families gave us books and tapes and recipes because they wanted us to live and they felt helpless. Although we appreciated the caring and love in those gifts, we reacted to a silent and probably unconscious message they carried: Did they really believe that we could cure ourselves by doing what the books and tapes described? Since we were frightened and fighting for our lives, it was difficult not to react with some resentment to the implied message that we weren't doing it right.

When Dorothy was diagnosed with breast cancer two years ago, she too found that some of the books and articles she read emphasized the individual's role in his or her illness in troublesome ways: "There are some things in the books that have a lot of validity, but there are a lot of threads that run through them that can undo someone. I think we need a lot more support to go through this process, [rather than] information that [makes us] feel guilty about having created our own illness. I had a person ask me once, 'Why do you think you gave yourself this disease?' and it's a good thing I didn't have a baseball bat. Who's going to give themselves cancer?"

In describing her feelings about the power of positive thinking, Martina had a very similar response to Dorothy's: "There's some truth in it, but put in the hands of some folks it's very damaging. I think to tell people with cancer they need to think positive thoughts and to make them feel guilty if what they're feeling is different—such as fear, anger, or any of those emotions—is to make things worse for them. Those emotions have to be expressed, they can't be repressed and do anybody any good."

Dorothy, sadly, also had to experience the confusion and helplessness those on the other side of the fence feel. Several years before she developed breast cancer, her nephew was diagnosed with cancer. At that time, she expressed an indirect belief that his attitude was not the right one for survival. In the face of her lack of control, she believed in the power of books and tapes to cure.

> I went out and bought maybe four or five books and tapes. That whole scenario came from this feeling of helplessness when someone that you love [is sick. His] resignation was so difficult for me to deal with until I finally realized that this was his disease and he had to make the choice of how he was going to deal with it. I needed to . . . let him know that I would support him in anything that he wanted but not to force [something] down his throat, which I was doing at first for my own benefit. I thought, "If I do this, maybe I'll help heal him." [Then] I realized that you can't do that.

As I mentioned earlier, Americans in the United States in the twentieth century hold some basic beliefs about life: that illness is caused by a known agent and can be cured; that if we follow the dictates of a healthy life-style, we are protected from sickness and even death; and that we can choose when and how we die. As cancer survivor Neil Fiore says in *The Road Back to Health: Coping with the Emotional Aspects of Cancer,* "The expectation of an understandable and controllable world is so deeply embedded in the modern mind that when horrific events occur we tend to attribute them to a logical, cause-effect relationship, rather than acknowledge that some things are still beyond our human understanding and the control of our technology. . . . As attempts to explain uncontrollable events, blame and self-blame are particularly damaging to one's ability to cope with cancer."

Nevertheless, many cancer survivors prefer to think they have created their own cancer rather than open themselves to the frightening possibility that their cancer is a random, meaningless event. As we struggle with cancer and mortality, we are coming to grips with the fact that certain key assumptions we have made about the world are myths—the myths of control, invulnerability, and immortality.

Where Did These Ideas Come From?

The notion of omnipotence is a child's fantasy that is nurtured by American popular culture. Jiminy Cricket promised us as children that magical thinking and rituals would get us what we wanted:

> When you wish upon a star,
> Makes no difference who you are.
> When you wish upon a star,
> Your dreams come true.

We still make wishes on birthday candles, put scraps of paper from fortune cookies in our wallets, read our horoscopes, and until it is proved otherwise, believe we can be and do anything by sheer force of want and will.

Wishful thinking is not restricted to positive outcomes. As children, we also believed we could cause misfortune and tragedy by our own spiteful thoughts or actions ("Step on a crack, break your mother's back"). As adults, we know there is no direct cause-and-effect relationship between our thoughts and what happens. Or do we? Katharine reflected on this as she talked about her cancer support group: "I finally realized that one reason it was important to me to hang in there with the people who were sick—even though I'm healthy now—was because I still feel guilty about not being with my parents when they died. I have this fantasy that if I had just been there and told them I loved them, they wouldn't have died." When Katharine examined her motives for staying in the group, she became conscious for the first time of her continuing childlike beliefs. She was then able to decide, with the awareness of an adult, whether to stay in the group. Her decision was no longer driven by the magical thinking of childhood.

Wishful thinking is at the core of creativity—but it is not a replacement for careful scientific thinking that clearly relates cause and effect. I think it is important that we keep examining our deepest and most primitive beliefs about the power of thoughts and actions. I believe that a diet of hamburgers and a cranky personality cannot create cancer. The picture of willing away cancer with good behavior and positive thoughts may be comforting, but it is a naïve fantasy.

This does not mean there is no relationship between your mind and your body. There is. And saying we do not have *ultimate* control does not mean we should be passive. If we give our bodies healthy food and our minds a sense of peace and happiness, we help our immune systems to function efficiently. However, this is not the same as saying we can prevent or cure serious illness or that we gave ourselves cancer because we didn't live right.

The Mind-Body Connection

There are many, many books written about the complex and mysterious relationship between mind and body. Scientific research on mind-body interaction has been conducted for a number of years, and conventional medicine now acknowledges that therapies and techniques that soothe the mind have a role in the physical health of patients.

Current thinking about the mind-body connection is that each influences the other. The mind is not separate from the body. Skeptics have only to remember the neck-, back-, or headaches we experience when we are worried or angry. Think of our language: "He's a real pain in the neck"; "I'm shouldering too many responsibilities now." We are whole organisms, and every part of our bodies, from cell to organ, influences and reacts to every other part. There is now agreement on the *fact* that mind and body are interdependent. But there is not yet a complete understanding of *how* the interaction occurs.

Given that the mind and the body are inextricably connected, it follows that treatment for a serious illness must take the whole person into account—mind and body. Physicians will treat the physical source of the problem—mending a bone that is broken; surgically removing, radiating, or chemically poisoning cancer cells. Techniques such as visualization and meditation will help to soothe the anxiety created by the broken bone, the tumor, or the treatment. Eating a low-fat balanced diet and participating in mild daily exercise also give our bodies what they need to function and reduce anxiety. All of these approaches work together to speed the healing process by bolstering our immune systems.

However, once again, a mind-body connection does not equal a cause and effect relationship. The mind can influence the body and vice versa. But the mind cannot create cancer nor can it cure it.

New Age Thinking: An Oversimplification

Research on the relationship between mind and body has been adapted by the New Age movement to produce an interpretation of illness in which we are able to control our destiny. Some New Age adherents have simplified a complex body of scientific research and spiritual beliefs into a set of prescriptive regulations.

According to these rules, illness is a lesson. We get sick so we can learn something important about ourselves. The message, therefore, is that we have given ourselves the disease, and if we don't learn the lesson the first time around, we will get sick again. This view vastly oversimplifies the intricate, complex, and still mysterious connection between mind and body.

One of the survivors interviewed is married to a woman who strongly believes in personal will. Her point of view helped him to examine and subsequently make positive changes in his life. However, at the time of his diagnosis, he also felt a burden of responsibility and guilt for having created his cancer. He reported:

> [My wife's] view is that people only die when they want to. And if you're sick, the question is, "What's this all about?" She's very rarely sick, and she has that view: she isn't sick

because she doesn't want to be, which is great if you're not sick. . . . So I had that to deal with. It was like, Am I copping out here? Am I doing something that I shouldn't be doing? Am I conflicted in some way that I'm not aware of? It was kind of difficult for me to deal with that part of it because I had the feeling I was failing her.

Eight years ago Martina was successfully treated for non-Hodgkin's lymphoma. Like many of the survivors, she believes that her state of mind played a part in her cancer but is angered by the idea that she could have caused it. "I had a very difficult time dealing with the people who have New Age interpretations of why people have cancer, because I think it's simplistic and offensive and it ticks me off. . . . It's not like I reject completely that there are psychological factors; I know there are. I just think it's too simplistic to say, 'Oh, you have cancer because you're whatever—fill in the blank.'"

Such oversimplification can lead people to assume that their friends gave themselves cancer to learn a lesson about themselves. These people innocently expect a rational reply to their questioning. Kat Duff, a New Age practitioner who found herself seriously ill, confesses, "I dread having to tell people I am sick, or still sick, because many respond with theories about what I did to make myself sick or suggestions of what I could do to get well—both of which just make me feel worse for being sick."

Research on the tendency for feelings of happiness, satisfaction, and purpose to impact our health positively has been oversimplified by the New Age movement to the prescription, "Cure your cancer with positive thinking." To those of us faced with the possibility of death, "think positive" becomes a tyrannical necessity. Having cancer and confronting mortality evokes many feelings, among them love for our lives and relationships and a will to remain alive. Yet equally valid and simultaneous responses are terror, anger, and depression. The popular insistence that we remain positive at all times or risk death is emotionally draining, produces unbearable guilt when we succumb to hopelessness, and denies us full expression of our experience.

Virginia, too, pointed out that overemphasizing positive thinking results in denying our painful feelings and that this stuffing down of unwanted feelings takes a lot of energy that we could otherwise expend more usefully. Denying our painful feelings also robs us of the deeply honest interactions with loved ones that are so fulfilling and sustaining. Virginia commented that, partly, "the New Age positive thinking is an attempt to get away from a self-blame orientation. [But] I think they just don't understand the full dynamics of how we function. [From the Jungian perspective], if you take something only of light, of positive, then you must negate the dark, the evil, and it's going to fester, build, be unacknowledged. The New Age overemphasizes the light and says you should not look at the dark, you should not look at negativity—as if anger or sadness is negative. They're just emotions."

Ken Wilber, seen by many as a New Age guru, found himself reevaluating his beliefs as his wife battled breast cancer. "The 'new age stance,' as I have come to see it, is largely defined by its narcissistic, grandiose, and omnipotent fantasies. And one of these grandiose fantasies is that, if we want to, we can 'visualize' disease as going away and the disease will simply go away. . . . Any careful examination of this field shows that the vast majority is shot through with magical or wish-fulfillment thinking. 'I can wish my disease away.' That's pure fixation on the magical level."

Many New Age writers are careful to distinguish between *healing* and *curing*. Healing draws on mental, spiritual, and emotional resources. We can strengthen them through techniques such as meditation, visualization, or journal writing. The goal of healing is to become more whole, comfortable with who we are, and satisfied with the way we are living our lives. Curing, in contrast, works to eliminate disease in the body; that is what mainstream medicine and physicians have to offer. We can experience healing whether we are physically cured of disease or not.

However, many readers pay little attention to this distinction because they want to hear what is going to cure them, what is going to get rid of their cancer forever, for sure. And even though self-help authors and speakers may define what they mean by healing, their descriptions of the results of visualization, diet, meditation, positive thinking, and love infusions do in fact infer *cure*. Dr. Bernie Siegel, for example, uses the term *healing* throughout his books but at the same time slips in unequivocal statements such as "Feelings are chemical and can kill or cure" and further blurs this critical distinction in his next statement: "As a doctor I believe it's my responsibility to help my patients use [feelings] to *cure and heal themselves*" (emphasis added).

Some New Age adherents twist the concept of responsibility into a position of blaming the victim (me and you), a stance that leads us into unproductive self-examination: Can I trust myself to do the best for myself or do I really hate myself so much that I am wishing illness and even death on myself? This line of thought undermines our ability to trust ourselves when we most need to believe that we are making wise decisions.

Your Illness as a Catalyst

If we stop blaming ourselves for our illness, we may even gain benefits from looking at our cancer in a creative way. Considering the type of cancer, its location, the timing of its appearance, *unrelated to cause or cure,* may provide us with some interesting personal insights. This act of "free association" may give us access to our deepest concerns, which may in turn act as a catalyst for making important changes in our lives.

For example, although Martina was clear that her dissatisfaction with her work did not create her non-Hodgkin's lymphoma, she also thought carefully about the symbolism she might draw from it and now believes she was in a spiritual crisis at that time. "If you want to do the New Age interpretation, it's interesting that the lymphoma was over my heart and that the work that I was doing didn't feel like it was coming from my heart at all. It was actually counter to everything that is important to me. . . . It was immediately clear to me that I didn't know what I was going to do when I got well, but it wasn't going to be what I had been doing."

Of course, Martina does not mean that her cancer occurred over her heart because her work did not feel as though it was coming from her heart. Instead, the cancer naturally caused her to focus on the part of her body it affected. She could have thought about what was happening there simply in terms of the damage caused by the cancer. Instead, she chose to think more deeply and symbolically about that part of her body. In this way, she found a means of recalling to herself the importance of her heart—not as a life-giving pump but as a symbol of the centrality of feelings and emotions in our lives, whether we acknowledge them or not. Through such metaphoric approaches, people can turn what they might perceive only as damage or loss into a useful insight. And of course, you do not have to have cancer or any other disease before you examine your heart or any other important physical part metaphorically and learn from that examination.

Virginia contemplated the meaning of the throat cancer she had thirty years ago. She stated that although she believes her cancer was a random event, "we can take something that may be random and look at what we get out of it in terms of learning. . . . In our family, we did not talk about dying [at times when a family member died] or emotions or the upsetness. We all pretended it didn't exist. And so I think I just was completely choked up. I stuffed down the feelings. [I was] unable to speak, unable to say what I thought, what I felt. The meaning [of my cancer] that made sense for me was that I wasn't allowed to tell my truth."

Virginia believes that her soul-searching about the meaning she might gain from her cancer led to her interest in psychology and her decision to become a psychotherapist.

Glenna's cancer, like Virginia's, affected her ability to speak. The meaning she created from having oral cancer also stimulated her to overcome old family prohibitions.

My cancer was a hole in my mouth, not a lump, and at first I joked that it was from all the times I put my foot in my mouth. But the sadder personal truth was that I hadn't put my foot in my mouth nearly enough. I had been taught that stoic silence was a virtue and that to say too much about myself was if not rude, indiscreet. I can hear my mother saying, "Young lady, that tone of voice will not do," every time I was angry, bossy, or whiny. With my cancer, I realized I'd never had permission to speak in all my voices but only the polite voice. I vowed that if I was so lucky as to have a voice after surgery, I would speak in all my varied voices.

Bente also found a metaphor in her cancer. She has devoted her professional life to spiritual examination and healing. For Bente, cancer of the cervix and uterus was symbolic of the devaluation she felt as a woman in a sexist society. She interpreted having cancer in "the physical center of her femininity" as symptomatic of the damage done to women. Exploring the meaning cancer held for her enabled Bente to reclaim herself and her creative powers. Although she had been working with these issues for years, Bente said that "cancer focused a spotlight on them." As she saw it, "A lost part of women came home to me," and the experience strengthened her—as a woman and a healer.

As I was working on this chapter, I thought hard about whether I had a metaphor for my cancer, a cancer that began on my skin and went inward. Although I could probably work that statement into something, I really do not have a metaphor. Some people do not, nor is it essential to have one.

Finding a Balance

Even though we may understand that there was probably no definitive cause of our cancer, at least not one within our control, we still want to do everything possible to keep it from returning. And that is the fine line we walk—staying aware that we did not cause our cancer while simultaneously practicing preventive measures. This is not as paradoxical as it sounds. The idea is to take good care of ourselves so we have resources to fight off disease. Specifically, we need to give our immune systems all the help we can.

Part of our being willing to *take* care of ourselves is to *feel* care. I remember feeling an overwhelming tenderness for my physical body when I was told I had cancer. I felt I had not fully appreciated it before it was in trouble, and I wanted to protect it from further harm. In the treatment of melanoma, the malignant mole is first cut out, and later, more skin around the area is removed. Fortunately, I had a good relationship with my surgeon. When I went in for the second surgery, I felt comfortable asking him to please talk to the area on my back he was cutting and to explain to it that it had done a great job of healing from the first surgery, but now he had to do more in order to help it. I didn't care if he thought I was nuts; I just wanted my body to know he and I cared about it.

When my cancer recurred two years later, all the lymph nodes in my right armpit were removed. Only one node was cancerous, but all the other nodes in the area were enlarged from fighting the disease. I wrote in my journal how sad I felt that those valiant nodes had to be sacrificed when they had been doing such a good job for me.

Living in a healthy way will not make us invulnerable to sickness and death. But it makes sense to take care of ourselves to promote our quality of life. Moreover, actively doing something keeps us from feeling that we are helpless and then giving up.

Sometimes we stumble on the fine line in the other direction. If we have no control over cancer, we may come to see no point to eating appropriately, exercising, and relaxing. The point is that although pessimism won't kill us, our feelings can lead to a state of depression. And depression does inhibit the immune system. Taking responsibility for ourselves is no *guarantee*, but it helps.

As a psychotherapist as well as a cancer survivor, Virginia has studied the relationship between individuals' psychological states and their health. She has used her insights to bring more playfulness into her life. She says: "I believe that any kind of thought we have impacts our soma [physical being] and that if you stay in the negative framework, you'll increase depression, you'll increase illness, you'll wear your body down. Since [a recent scare of recurrence], I made a very conscious decision to change my life entirely. . . . I'm going to have fun." Virginia just bought herself something she had always wanted: a beautiful new green four-by-four car that makes her laugh every time she drives it.

Taking responsibility for keeping ourselves as healthy as possible also gives us some peace of mind in the limbo of life after cancer. Dr. Irvin Yalom is a psychiatrist who has worked with many cancer patients. He believes that "cancer, perhaps more than any other disease, fosters a sense of helplessness— patients feel unable to exert any personal control over their condition . . . patients with cancer feel they can do nothing but wait—wait until the next cancer cell pops up somewhere in the body." If we take an "active stance" in our own care, we feel more in control of the uncontrollable.

We search for an explanation of why we got cancer in the first place so that we know what to do to prevent its recurrence. As survivors, however, we now understand the trap of omnipotence and know we did not create nor can we cure our cancer. We begin to understand that an unrelenting will to stay positive at all costs, to live right and be perfect, robs us of the chance to be ourselves, warts and all. It puts the emphasis on "doing life right" rather than on living. Cancer has forced us to evaluate our lives and understand what is important to us. Once we know what is important, we can begin to do those things that make us feel glad to be alive. Then we are no longer sidestepping the dance of limbo but participating fully in it.

7

Social Dancing After Cancer

"Spiders give me the creeps," said Emily, a friend from childhood who was visiting for a few days about a year after my surgery. "If I see one at home, I pull out the vacuum and suck up everything in sight. Once I even did it in the middle of the night when I woke up and saw a spider on the ceiling." "Oh no! It's very bad luck to kill spiders in a house," said Barbara, another friend, who lives up the road. "Just put them outside on a broom, but never kill them, or you'll have bad luck."

The next morning, Emily said to me, "There was a huge spider in the bathroom sink, and everyone was asleep so I couldn't ask for help, and I was afraid to kill the spider after what Barbara said. So I held my breath and gritted my teeth and picked it up with a Kleenex and put it on the floor. If anything ever happened to you, I would always wonder if it was because I killed that spider, and I would never be able to forgive myself."

LISA

This simple episode has stayed with me because of Emily's spontaneous expression of her love and worry for me and because of all that was unspoken. As I thought about it later, I decided Emily was expressing her feelings of helplessness and her wish to be able to affect the uncontrollable. I knew she thought about my cancer frequently. Since my recurrence, she had telephoned me more often. We never talked about this directly, but each time she telephoned the thought would race through my mind that she called because she knew I might die from my cancer. I'm not saying that every time she picked up the phone she said to herself, "I'd better call Lisa because she could die." But I believe that the threat of losing me forever made her consciously value our long friendship.

I noticed that my brother, my cousin, and other friends were also making contact with me more frequently than before. My cancer reminded all of us to actively appreciate each other now. At the same time, my relationship with the man in my life felt wildly unstable, and some friends had stopped calling. At some point, I realized that nearly all my relationships were undergoing change. In retrospect, I can see that it would have been bizarre if they remained the same, since they and I had all been through a traumatic and transforming experience.

As Glenna and I have discussed at length in this book, most survivors are changed by having had cancer. We are confronted with difficult questions and feel unprotected. Eventually, however, our internal drama loses intensity, and our attention turns outward. We then see that because we are different, relationships with people we care about are altered as well. Our relationships are the place in which all our new ways of being and understanding are played out. Some relationships end; others deepen. As we learn to live in the limbo of life after cancer, we must learn how to dance with others. This is not always easy.

Fear Can Cripple the Dance

The need to deal with fear of death and loss is one issue that is common to all kinds of relationships. Yet each of us has his or her own level of tolerance for these feelings and ways of coping with the discomfort. In every relationship, we must come to terms with that fear if the relationship is to continue.

Dancing to Different Beats

In the beginning, coming to terms with fear is difficult because it is experienced by us and by those we love at different times. During diagnosis and treatment, most of us feel optimistic and in charge. After the first rush of fear and despair, we put all our energy into coping and recovery. Our self-centered focus helps get us through the crisis. During this time, we often find our families and friends are more realistic about the situation and more in contact with their fear than we are.

When Glenna told her friend Nanine that she had cancer, Nanine had an intuitive optimistic sense that Glenna would be fine. However, at work the following day, she told a doctor friend that Glenna had oral cancer. He blanched, sat Nanine down, and told her that if Glenna lived she would be lucky and that she was probably not going to have a mouth/face/jaw. Nanine felt as if she had been hit by a ton of bricks and was enormously torn about what to say to Glenna. Did Glenna know how bad this could be? Should she tell her? How could she comfort her? At a time when Nanine needed most to talk with her friend, she felt she could not.

Experts such as Merle H. Mishel and her research team suspect that during early phases of cancer diagnosis and treatment, a full awareness of the danger "may be blunted . . . because the patient is preoccupied with the experience of enduring treatment." When the rigors of treatment are behind us, however, there is both time and energy to face the large, unanswerable question: Will I live or will I die?

At the end of treatment our partners, friends, and family assume the crisis is past and things will return to normal. Just as they are breathing sighs of relief, we are emerging from our trauma-induced numbness. As we slowly absorb the reality of what we have been through, fears of recurrence begin to emerge. But at first, we do not understand these fears, nor do we know how to manage them. Our anxieties can drive those closest to us nuts.

For a while, I worried that every wheeze, sneeze, cough, and blink was metastatic cancer. Even I got tired of hearing myself, but I couldn't stop. These fears were very real to me. My boyfriend got the lion's share of my worrying. He was supportive, but when pushed, said he didn't understand why I worried myself over something hypothetical, something he strongly believed would never happen.

A crisis in relationships can come at this point, when communication around the issue of cancer and fear is difficult and unclear. Our fears are coming up at different times. Our friends say, "What's the matter with you? You should be feeling wonderful—you're well; you don't have cancer any more." We say, "You don't understand what I've been through," and feel isolated. Neither they nor we know enough to articulate what is really going on. For us, it is recognizing our vulnerability for the first time, facing the idea that we really can't control anything, being terrified we will die before we are ready. For them, it is not wanting to be reminded of how helpless they felt when we were sick and how afraid they were we might die. They just want to put those old fears behind them and may become impatient if we persist in talking about them.

When You Can't Even Hear the Music

When relationships are complex and interdependent, as they are in a marriage or a business partnership, the fear of loss is so intolerable that the survivor's partner may literally become deaf to the topic of cancer.

During Glenna's treatment, her husband was completely present, emotionally and physically. Afterward, Glenna noticed that he changed the subject every time she talked about her cancer-related fears. When she had a scheduled medical checkup or a recurrence scare (as happened twice), he suddenly went out of town on business. He seemed to have no awareness of what he was doing. Fortunately, Glenna knew him well enough to understand that he simply could not bear even a theoretical discussion of death after he had come so close to losing her. If

Glenna had died, her husband would not only have lost her physical presence in his life; his daily life, home, work, and sense of identity would also have been irrevocably changed. It is no wonder that he did not want to hear about her fears or be around for the results of her checkups! He—like almost anyone in his position—needed to avoid his fears of loss. With both disappointment and humor, Glenna accepted his position and called her friends when her fears needed voicing. She says now, "The only reason I was able to laugh about this was because I understood that we were out of sync, and because he had been both so present and also openly terrified of losing me [during treatment] that I knew his behavior [later] was to take care of him, not to hurt me."

I had a similar experience. From the time my recurrence was diagnosed until I returned to work, my business partner, Donna, and I talked on the phone frequently. Donna was worried for me and wanted to know what was happening and how I felt. When I decided to take a three-month sabbatical, she was totally supportive and willing to handle the business alone for the time I was gone. She also figured out how we could manage this financially. At the end of three months, we both expected that I would be energized, back to normal, and eager to dig into work again. I wasn't. I was smack in the middle of anxiety, depression, and vulnerability. The only thing I knew for sure was that I didn't know what I wanted. We had many emotional meetings over how to restructure the business to satisfy our increasingly different needs. We finally brought in a business counselor to help us sort things out.

During this meeting, I explained that my cancer had returned, I had taken time off after my surgery, and I was not sure what I wanted to do with my life. I did know I didn't want to spend all of my time and energy on work, even though I cared very much about the business and about my relationship with Donna. The counselor said immediately, "You're dealing with some very difficult existential issues right now. What are the chances your cancer could come back?" I explained that there was a 50 percent chance it would return. Donna was completely shocked. I had assumed she had known this and understood what I was grappling with. Like Glenna's husband, she probably found it just too difficult to contemplate the complexity of her loss—personally and for our business—if anything happened to me. (Conversely, I may have failed to mention the odds since I didn't want to think about them either!)

As is characteristic of our relationship, we never again referred to this discussion. But because we had talked openly about *why* each of us needed to change our contract, we were able to work out a new agreement that satisfied both of us.

Survivors' relationships with their families of origin are also complex, and communicating about fears and losses within families may be exquisitely difficult. As a child, Glenna had both counted on and dreaded her mother's habit of bringing up the uncomfortable things Glenna was avoiding talking about. After her cancer diagnosis, she expected this same behavior from her mother.

> I had told my mother of my diagnosis and impending surgery on the phone. I was eager to see her: I wanted her to hold me, rock me like a baby, and share my fears. I wanted her to open my mouth, look at that nasty cancer, and curse it. When I arrived to see her, Mother was breezy, busy with packing for a long-scheduled trip, chattering on about her itinerary. I waited patiently, then impatiently. She never mentioned my cancer. Finally my aunt, with whom Mother was traveling, asked about my surgery. We talked briefly, and my normally reserved aunt expressed her tender concern. Mother searched for her eyedrops. I was speechless and finally managed a goodbye. As we parted, Mother hugged me and said, "I just know everything will come out fine." I left reeling. I had wanted my mommy, and in her place I'd found a self-absorbed stranger.

The possibility of Glenna's death was too horrible for her mother to think about, so she didn't. Her preoccupation with packing her bags was one way not to think the unthinkable, feel the unfeelable.

Impossible Expectations
and Magical Allies

Under ordinary circumstances, it is easy to have unrealistic expectations of a partner, friend, or family member. Once cancer enters our lives, we feel vulnerable and want unconditional understanding and support. However, if this support was not an element of our relationships before cancer, it is unlikely to develop after cancer. Much like Glenna, I wanted my mommy. But because my mother is dead, I turned to my aunts. In the back of my mind, I hoped that they would appear at my bedside to tell me how much they loved me. They didn't, for any number of practical reasons, but also because such behavior would have been uncharacteristic.

Before cancer, we may have accepted the limitations of a relationship. But while we are coping with so many losses, it is especially painful to experience our disappointment when a close relationship cannot deliver. Many of the survivors interviewed said that in retrospect, they had expectations that might have been unrealistic.

The immediate crisis of cancer tends to bring out the best in us—at first. The trauma of diagnosis leaves our emotions raw, and it seems easy to be open with each other about our love and fears. Our hopeful expectations may naturally be that this closeness, which often reminds couples of their courtship or early domestic life, will continue. What often happens is that the fear of loss kicks in and an important person in our lives pulls back. The pattern is reminiscent of the phases we follow in limbo: we start on a high where everything is simple and clear, and then we tumble into a place that feels lonely and unfamiliar. Our intimate relationships may parallel this process, and we may suffer disillusionment with the people we counted on most.

Charlotte's mother had died from cancer when Charlotte was seventeen. The way her father took care of her mother created Charlotte's unconscious expectations of her husband when she developed breast cancer: "The one thing I really regret is that I can't get the support from him I really would like to. My father was one hundred percent behind my mother and loved her even more. And I thought that was going to be the case [in my marriage], and for one month after my diagnosis, we had a marvelous relationship. It was almost like when we first met. And I felt warmth. And one month later, it was gone."

Although Charlotte and her husband experienced an initial intimacy, her husband then pulled away, probably because his fear became too strong. What made his retreat particularly disillusioning for Charlotte was her expectation, formed in adolescence, about how husbands are supposed to behave.

Sometimes our culture promotes certain romanticized expectations about relationships. One of these notions is that adversity strengthens love. As Ellen reflected on her marriage during her cancer, she described having certain expectations that were not met. "It was very shattering to have us not become closer in crisis, because I had really always believed that love was born from crisis and that crisis was unifying. . . . That [the crisis] didn't pull us closer together [is something I] sometimes still cry about."

Because we also have high and often unrealistic expectations of our families of origin, there is the potential for feeling devastated. Dorothy tells a sad story about her sister, on whom she relied and whom she had expected to help her through her illness. "I grew up with my sister and was always at her house. She's quite a bit older than me and was like a second mother. I thought [she] would be my biggest support, but it just became too much for her and she never came to see me and barely phoned me. That was very upsetting for me. It was like being deserted."

Although Dorothy could cite compelling reasons for her sister's behavior (her sister's son had died of cancer seven months earlier and the sister had been diagnosed with cancer as her son was dying), her sense of abandonment was real and unassuaged by an intellectual understanding. At the same time, Dorothy understood the role her expectations had played in the situation. "I realized that I had to come to terms with what kind of relationship I was going to have with my sister and her husband from this point on, and that took a lot of soul-searching on my part. Just realizing that my expectations for her and her husband had to totally change for me to start feeling better—that was very hard because a lot of times expectations are built up around our family."

A common variation on the theme of expectations is the belief in a magical ally, a "special person," as Dorothy said, "whoever it might be, who can help you through the whole thing. Sometimes maybe it's going to be a family member that you're really close with, or a lover. It can probably take different forms, this special person."

Even if we do not believe that love conquers all, we wish that it could. The wish to have our wounds kissed and magically healed is one more example of the regression to childish thinking that is part of any illness. That wish to kiss and restore what we have lost is a regressed solution to an intolerable problem. When we love someone with cancer, we can neither cure the cancer nor be indifferent to its outcome, so we are left powerless and dependent. Those are feelings from early childhood, and as in childhood, we believe in magic.

Although Dorothy expressed a flexibility about who fills the magical ally role, most of us expect this special role to be willingly filled by our mate. If she or he is not suited to the task, we are sorely disappointed, and irreparable damage may be done to the relationship. If we do not have a mate, we feel cheated of the possibility of rescue, even though that possibility is unrealistic.

The need for a magical ally was something I experienced strongly after my cancer and was eventually able to recognize but not change. From the day the tumor under my arm was found, I developed an intense dependency on the man I loved. The only time I felt really safe, when the tension in my body could melt, was when he was holding me. Just having him nearby calmed me. Talking with friends, which I did often, helped me a lot but did not give me that sense of physical comfort and relief. When my crisis was past and my fear was less evident, I still became very anxious when I was separated from him. I had somehow decided that he could keep me safe, even from death.

He willingly participated in the belief that he could save me. He said: "Every time you had a close call, . . . I pulled you back, and you felt that if I hadn't pulled you back you could have died." Although he wanted to be my magical ally, he knew there were limits on what was possible, so playing the protector raised in him conflicting feelings of both willingness and obligation. When we talked about this recently, he said, "All of a sudden, I realized I had to be there, both emotionally and materially, for anything that you might need. And giving that [support] became central to our relationship. I enjoyed being a caretaker for you, and I knew that I *had* to follow through."

However, a partner's willingness to fill the role of magical ally may place the relationship in jeopardy. When such powerful and largely unconscious forces are at play in relationships, both partners and cancer survivors are simply damned if they don't and damned if they do. Providing the kind of support that gets someone through the whole experience is physically and emotionally draining. To be the object of such profound dependence can be frightening; to recognize that one is that dependent is more frightening still. Denial of their dependence is one reason that many cancer patients are genuinely incapable of appreciating the toll all the supportive actions take on their magical allies. For the patient, surviving cancer is a full-time preoccupation. Appreciating the sacrifices made by another, especially when the other is healthy and unharmed by invasive treatments, is simply impossible. If the magical ally ends up feeling underappreciated, retaliation is virtually inevitable. To complicate matters further, the magical ally may not appreciate the magnitude of her or his own efforts or their cost.

Renegotiating Intimate Relationships

The lasting effects of having had cancer may disrupt intimate relationships in many ways. Many couples find their normal flow of emotions thrown out of sync. At the very time one part-

ner begins to feel more confident of survival, the other is overcome with fears of death. When one is ready to put the experience behind him or her, the other suddenly needs to talk about
the meaning of it all. Sometimes the difference in timing can
be useful because one person is up while the other is down. Frequently, however, when the ebb and flow of thoughts and feelings doesn't match, couples who are accustomed to being in
sync can feel distressed. For those who have difficulty communicating in ordinary times, adjusting to life after cancer can be
an overwhelming task.

Glenna and Curtis were normally very much in sync with
each other. However, when Curtis's father died six months
after Glenna's cancer, they found their individual needs at cross-
purposes. Glenna was still very vulnerable and determined to
take care of herself. For Curtis, nearly losing Glenna, knowing
she was still at risk, and then losing his father was almost more
than he could bear. In his grief, he directed a lot of his anger
at Glenna. For the first time in their relationship, she said no,
this will not do. And they went together to a therapist, also for
the first time. They needed a third person to help them learn
how to deal with loss and grief without hurting each other and
their relationship. The new ways they learned to communicate
around these hard issues have held them in good stead during
subsequent losses.

One reason that a relationship may be forced to change is
that the customary balance of power has shifted. Think of all
the ways cancer can change us. If our career has been disrupted,
our earning power diminished, our ability to do things for ourselves and others compromised, our appearance altered, our
energy sapped (to name only a few of the possibilities), we have
lost some of our power. If we feel stronger, more aware of our
own feelings and needs, more deeply connected to those we
love, and clearer about our priorities, this increase in personal
power will also tip the old balance.

Sometimes it is not us but our partner who undergoes the
most transformation. To the degree that either person in a relationship is different because of the experience, the relationship,

particularly if it is a very close one, will inevitably go through some change.

Charlotte felt her cancer had given her a new strength that her husband had not yet adjusted to. "With my cancer, I've gotten much stronger, and he hates to see that. I think he wants me to be the way I was when we were married, when I came to this country. I knew English, but not the way I do now. I was so helpless, and he thrived in the role that he had. He's taken out of his role now by me being much stronger because of what happened to me."

There Are No Perfect Families

In the first sentence of *Anna Karenina*, Tolstoy says, "All happy families resemble one another; each unhappy family is unhappy in its own way." In my experience, there are no perfectly happy families. All have some unhappiness. In the language of family therapy, all have some dysfunction. Whatever is dysfunctional in any family will probably become painfully apparent in the face of cancer. Just when we need the best our family has to offer, we sometimes get the worst as well. With the crisis over, we may need to renegotiate the terms of our family relationships, just as we have renegotiated other important relationships in our lives. Because of the history that family members have with each other, this renegotiation can be stubbornly difficult.

Cancer seems to bring out magical thinking in spades. Not only do we place impossible expectations of protection on our partners, we also expect our families of origin to respond in ways that belong to fantasy. Because family is family, we usually expect even more from family members than we do from anyone else. And they expect more from themselves.

This is not to say that families don't come through. Both Glenna and I got support from our brothers that surpassed our expectations. My brother, John, was the first person I called when I got the news about the tumor in my lymph node. He flew to be with me for the days before, during, and after my hospital stay and gave me the reassurance of his presence as well as the practical help of marketing, cooking, and driving me around. This was a reversal of roles for us, since I am the big sister and have always been the caretaker. When John thought back to those early days of my cancer, he said, "I suddenly found myself in a different position. Instead of being the little brother, I felt responsible for you. I'd never been in that position before, caring for you and basically looking out for you. It felt good. I was very scared, but I was glad that I was able to be there to support you."

On the day Glenna was waiting for the pathologist to call with the results of her biopsy, her brother, Ed, called to see how she was. "I'm coming over," he said. "Oh, I'm okay, you don't need to do that," Glenna told him. But Ed appeared and held Glenna's hand when the phone call came. And he stayed to hold Curtis's as well when he got home to hear the news.

Most families have unspoken rules about showing and sharing feelings, and any rules about hiding true feelings—especially fears—persist in the face of cancer. A customary prohibition against talking about feelings may become even stronger if family members believe that any discussion of cancer will upset the cancer patient. Although Norm lived in the same town as his parents when his cancer was diagnosed, five years later he remarked, "I still to this day don't know how [my family] dealt with it. People tell me that my mom was worried. I'm sure she was, but she never really let on. Nobody really let on."

There was a rule in my family about not sharing feelings, which I broke when I got cancer. For both me and my brother, it was necessary to talk about it, and John remarked on how different this was for us: "When Mom had cancer and Pop was ill, the way with all of us was not to talk about it. But in your case, it was quite different—we could talk about it, and you wanted to talk about it. I found that that took a lot of the fear out of it. I was able to pay more attention to it and not to push it aside."

Because of this family rule of not talking about illness, I believed that my beloved godmother, a second mother to me after my mother died, had either forgotten about my cancer after a year or really did not love or care about me. Then one evening, I mentioned something to her about my work on this book and the anxieties it brought up in me. She said with great relief, "I was so afraid you weren't taking the cancer seriously—you never talk about it!" How sad that we had both been thinking about the same thing but neither of us thought to break the silence. It is worth noting that we never talked about it again, but now I know that is because of the strength of our family rule, not because my godmother doesn't care.

Ann was very private about discussing her cancer and shared her thoughts only with her husband. She would have liked to be able to communicate more directly with her grown children but didn't feel it was possible.

> If I did [talk with others], it would be to my children, and I can't do it, mainly because I become too emotional and they do, too. For instance, last summer I put a box of dishes together, and I brought it down to our daughter. I didn't ask if she wanted them or not. I just brought them because I realized she could use them, and so I left them in her utility room. They came back from their vacation, and I said, "If you don't want them, just give them away. I don't need them." And she said, "Are you trying to tell me something?" I said, "No." She said, "Would you tell me when something is wrong?" And I said, "I promise you, I will."

Occasionally cancer is the catalyst for creating a more authentic and caring communication with family members. Norm's story has a bittersweet ending. Several years after his recovery, his mother became ill and had brain surgery. In the hospital just before she died, Norm was able to talk to his mother in a way he had never before been able to, and he attributes this change to his own experience with cancer. "We said everything we needed to say, back and forth in a couple of conversations that were almost otherworldly. We had this moment together when we just exchanged these words. My

family doesn't do that. That's what makes this experience
very special. And so, even in the moment of incredible grief
loss, it was a treasure. I wouldn't have had that experience
hadn't had my cancer."

Relationships can also change in small ways. Barbara and her
parents developed a new habit of telling each other, "I love you"
frequently. "Once you've been through something like that,
there's always a closeness. That level of caring dissipates, but we
all still say, 'I love you,' to each other when we talk to each other.
My parents . . . hardly ever did that before. It scared them!"

Dancing with Your Friends

When we need relief from the intensity of our intimate and
family relationships, friends are there for fun and for the no-
strings-attached support we may be craving. I had developed
many close friendships in my graduate program, and I had also
learned how to dance. The joy of moving my body to music
with people I trusted and cared about released me from my
tendency to be too much in my head. Twice a year at graduation, the community of students, faculty, staff, graduates, and
their families come together to celebrate. Part of this celebration is dancing to music from a hodgepodge of eras—swing,
rock, rap, rock and roll. Dancing in this community of friends
has never failed to reconnect me with my feelings and with all
that is good about life.

Several research studies have found that cancer patients are
typically more satisfied with the support they get from friends
than with the support of family members. As documented by
Nancy Waxler-Morrison and her colleagues, family disappoints,
but friends deliver. Friends are under no obligation to be there
for us. They do not live with us, and they do not experience
the "shoulds" that accompany blood ties. When their fear is
strong, they can choose not to be with us. They are often able
to give more with no strings attached because they are free to
come and go according to their needs, feelings, and schedules.

They can get the space that partners cannot take without raising feelings of abandonment. With friends, there are fewer of the expectations that can be so devastating to other, more intimate relationships.

Both Glenna and I and most of the women survivors who were interviewed received an infusion of love from their friends at the time of their diagnosis and treatment that caught them off guard. (Perhaps significant is the fact that none of the men interviewed talked about friends.) Ellen experienced the way her friends pulled together as "a gift." "The support was unbelievable. I still have cards from people and remember the fruit packages and visits and everything. It was just incredible, knowing who my friends were that I was deeply linked with and how they were there for me."

Charlotte has coffee with a group of friends every Thursday morning at her local café. The morning of her mastectomy, she said, "I went down there with my niece because I wanted to show her the café, and none of my friends was there. Many of them are Catholics, and they all went to mass and prayed for me while I was . . . waiting there for them. . . . And then they all showed up at the hospital. I thought that was fantastic, and I thrived from it."

All the women survivors said they couldn't have done it without their friends. Dorothy was quite specific about how they helped her. "When I went through this process, I realized what was real important was my friends just checking in. And the check-ins kind of gave me the strength to say, 'Okay, I can get through this. I've got people out there who care about me, and I can do it.'. . . Support from my friends was what really helped me get through as well as I did."

Socorro mentioned the importance of reciprocity in friendships. "Did it surprise me that all my friends and family rallied to my side? No, because I really demand a lot of my friends when I'm healthy, and I give a lot, too. I don't know if I expected it, but it didn't surprise me. I needed it, and they just gave."

When Glenna had the tracheostomy tube in her throat, she had a lot of trouble sleeping and was afraid to be alone in the hospital at night. Her friends just divvied up the nights so she always had someone to stay with her. She didn't spend one night alone until the tube was out. Several of her friends confessed they were more concerned for Curtis than for her. She was grateful because she knew he needed support. It was very sensitive of them not to neglect him. They recognized that this was as big a deal for him as for her.

All of the women interviewed also said that in the aftermath, some friendships had dropped away, but many friendships had deepened. Friends valued each other more consciously than they had before because of the awareness that something could happen to either one of them to cut short their time together. My very close friend Jane moved abroad with her family for two years not long after my surgery. Her fear for me and knowledge that if anything happened to me she could not be there immediately were among her chief regrets about leaving the United States. Possibly because we remembered my cancer, we wrote each other faithfully and frequently during those two years.

During the crisis of cancer, most survivors found that they went through an instant reprioritizing of the elements of their lives and that friends and relationships invariably came out on top. It takes soul-shaking trauma to remind us that meeting work deadlines and cleaning the house are meaningless in comparison with nurturing our relationships.

Dorothy talked about this in terms of the quality of the time she now spends with her friends. "I think I evaluate my friends and how I choose to spend my time. Before, I had a variety of concentric circles that went out, and sometimes I chose to spend more than I really should on [the] very outer ring, which I don't do now. I try to spend it with the rings that are much closer in and are more significant to me . . . I choose to spend my time maybe a little more carefully."

A Place Where People Understand: Support Groups

People who know us well, those in our inner circle, have shared in our journey with cancer. Some of us have also attended a cancer support group when we felt we needed a regular time in which to learn more about living with cancer. Having had cancer is an experience that sets us apart from others. The reality of death, the possibility of dying before we were ready, and our lack of say in the matter was shoved right in our faces. We live with that memory and with the knowledge that if it happened once, it could happen again. At any time. We understand that if it isn't cancer, it *will* be something else. Contrary to our previous beliefs, we will not be around forever.

Learning the Territory of Recovery

We can talk about these feelings with others, but time and again, survivors said they felt that friends and family could not understand survivors' feelings completely. For these reasons, many of us seek out a cancer support group to help us move through the crisis of cancer and learn the new territory of recovery. One of the most immediate functions of a support group is to provide the sympathy of others who have been there too. I joined a group of about seven melanoma patients and survivors and their partners six months after my surgery. It was one of many active steps I could take to care for myself.

Dorothy attended a group for women with breast cancer and said that "the bad part was getting cancer; the good part was meeting some incredibly wonderful, courageous women [with whom I] formed a very strong bond." The group gave Dorothy the important gift of feeling understood. "There was someone to talk with there that knew exactly what you were going through . . . family and friends can empathize, but they can't really know the fear of when you have heard that you have cancer and basically what you're looking at is, 'Gee, I wonder how much longer I have.' And it's hard to know that, unless you have been in that place, so . . . I was very fortunate in getting this group."

It can be difficult to talk about our fears and feelings with people we love because we want to protect them. They may also be tired of hearing our worries. In a support group, we don't have to be concerned about that. We don't have to protect anyone. We can talk about our thoughts about death without holding back and with an immediacy that is impossible in most social groups. That kind of sharing creates powerful bonding and provides relief.

Jeannette also commented on the fears that talk of cancer and death can stir up for other people.

> I think that some things are difficult to share with other people—mostly because I wouldn't want to burden someone else or [because] they may be avoiding facing certain things themselves. They may also feel uncomfortable because they're unable to offer real help or reassurance, and I would end up reassuring them. I think there can be an intellectual understanding, there can be a certain amount of empathy, but only someone who's in the same situation as you are really knows. I mean there are certain things [that] don't even have to be said. You just know, and they just know.

Most of the time, we engage in denial of our own deaths. If we did not, we could not function. As my friend Jane said, "Life would be like one long therapy session." For the most part, we are successful in our denial. However, just because we would like to forget about our cancer and our mortality doesn't mean they are going to disappear.

Groups provide a safe place to talk about our fear and anxiety. They can act as appropriate containers for these feelings, a way of bringing them under control. Norm has been meeting monthly with his support group for five years. He says that, this way, once a month he thinks about his cancer, and then he can forget it for the rest of the month. Moreover, being in the group is a reminder to him to appreciate his health and not ever take life for granted.

Brian had a similar response to being in a group.

> The first year after my diagnosis was filled with ups and downs, especially downs. Moderate elation would fill part of a day, followed by severe depression until bedtime. These ups and

downs were annoying to me and must have been difficult for
people around me. The experiences and discussions with the
other members of the group have given me a more reasonable,
middle-of-the-road perspective on being a melanoma victim.
I feel a tendency to naturally alternate between not thinking
about melanoma and thinking too much about it. The group
tends to act as a governor on the ups and downs.

Another important function of a group is to normalize our
feelings. Partners and friends, no matter how caring and per-
ceptive they are, cannot do this as well if they have not "been
there." Learning that our feelings are normal and shared by
others is especially valuable when we are learning to live in
limbo. When we can see that all the others in the group worry
that their cancer will return, do a minor freak-out when they
get a cold or a headache or a pimple, feel anxious before a regular checkup, and have times of feeling depressed and out of
control, we can say, "Oh, so I'm not crazy after all." That is not
only an enormous relief; it is also one less thing to worry about.

Being with people who share our deepest feelings decreases
the sense of isolation and disorientation that plagues us at different times. This experience of isolation isn't quite the same
thing as not being understood by the people we are closest to.
It has more to do with our new deep and frightening understanding that we have no choice but to live our own lives in our
own skins, come what may. Loving and communicating with
others fully and completely cannot alter our knowledge that we
are actually alone in the world. This realization can be devastating. When we first wake up in limbo, our environment,
friends, and daily routine are all the same, yet we feel in some
way separate from everything. Fortunately, waking up in limbo
does not last long, and verbalizing these feelings in a support
group can help us understand them. Ellen comments on this
process: "I'm different. There's a sadness that there's a part of
me that very few people really understand . . . a private part of
me. I'd love to be better at communicating with people so they
can understand this big part of me. . . . It's definitely a bond

that I find with other cancer survivors, just to be able to talk about it. . . . It's a real deep understanding that someone else has gone through a similar feeling and similar changes."

Learning About Death

There is one reason I have continued to attend my support group that I am uncomfortable telling to very many people. The group meetings are rare and special opportunities to learn about dying. Since I joined my group two years ago, two people have died from the same cancer I had. Seeing what the disease is capable of doing shook me to my toes and has more than once sent me into weeklong anxieties for myself. But being part of their experience was also an opportunity I would not have traded. I felt great love and admiration for both Nancy and Narayan as they fought their disease and alternated between optimism, disbelief, anger, fear, and acceptance.

Because I was supported by the others in the group, I was able to put myself in their shoes as they talked about their feelings and start to explore what I believe about life and death. I realized that each of us has a different view of what happens when we die, and these views have given me much to think about. I do believe that dying is part of living, and being a peripheral part of Nancy's and Narayan's deaths has helped me to understand how that is possible.

Brian also spoke about the impact of the deaths of support group members on his thoughts and feelings about his own inevitable death. "I had not yet really learned about the process of dying. . . . I have always wanted to die with dignity, but I didn't yet know how. The intellectual side of me was challenged to learn more about how to die in a way that would leave everyone with good memories of me. These memories may be the entire summation of my existence here on earth. . . . I don't believe I am becoming callous through exposure to dying; I may be more accepting of the natural progression of things and more confident that I can participate with friends who will understand."

Brian's acceptance of the natural progression of things and of sharing this with friends is the essence of social dancing in limbo. Once we have learned some dance steps on our own, we put them together in a pattern so we can move around the floor with the people we like and trust, the people we love. As I did with my friends at graduation celebrations, we can feel the joy of moving spontaneously in this new world.

8

Making Sense of Life

*An old friend died. I had always found him hard to take, but
my husband was devoted to the man, and I cared about his wife.
So we sat in a junior college auditorium in rural Texas while
associates paid him tribute. A famous woman stepped to the
podium. She is a gifted orator, but she laid her speech aside
to say what was on her mind. Our friend had self-destructed.
As a politician, his public policy had been thoughtful and
decent. His personal life was not. She spoke these sad facts with
wit and without malice. Then she delivered her eulogy. It was
fine, but it was her honesty that moved me.*

GLENNA

Sitting in that college auditorium, I reflected on the dead
man. For better or for worse, he had lived out the mis-
matched parts of himself. When his heart condition was diagnosed, he refused to talk about it. He rejected all recommended
treatments and refused to change his ways. He continued to
drink and to chop his own wood and died the way he wanted
to—at his home, chopping firewood. I could not begrudge
him. However, it was the woman who set her text aside to tell
the truth who called me to account.

It had been ten years since the tumor grew at the base of
my tongue. I had not known if I would be able to speak after

141

the surgery, and it had not mattered. I wanted to live. But I promised myself that if I lived, and if I could still talk, I would tell my truth.

Telling the truth as I know it has proved harder than I expected. Forming words with my scarred tongue is relatively easy. Honesty is not. I slip into old ways, saying what is expected in place of what I mean. Then someone dies, and I face the hard truth. My days are numbered. Not because I had cancer. I have survived that. But as a cancer survivor, I carry within me the certain knowledge that I will die, that I am alive today, and that I have a promise to keep.

This chapter is about recreating our lives after we have been touched by death. Nearly all those Lisa and I interviewed believed that surviving cancer had changed their lives—forever and for the better. At some point, those of us who have survived cancer stop wondering why it happened. We get over the posttreatment letdown. We tolerate our fears of recurrence in the full knowledge that there is no sure cure. Our relationships are renewed on current terms. Life goes on.

While our preoccupation with cancer fades, our awareness of mortality remains. That heightened awareness guides our lives, whether we recognize it or not. It creates anxiety, but it also reminds us that we are alive. Our time on earth is short and precious. This is the stuff of great art and trite greeting cards. Only a writer of Franz Kafka's perverse gifts can get away with stating the obvious, "The meaning of life is that it stops." When we use a brush with death to refocus our lives in more authentic and meaningful ways, we are making the best of the situation, to be sure, but we are not romanticizing our misfortune. Cancer is not glamorous. Surviving cancer is neither romantic nor heroic. It is our good fortune, and it is forever part of our lives. We may feel stronger for having endured the trials, or we may feel more vulnerable. Probably we feel both, on alternate days or even at the same time. Sometimes we know that "sadder but wiser" is a cliché because it is true.

This chapter is not an inspirational greeting card. It is an admission that life is difficult. If we accept Longfellow's observation that "into each life some rain must fall," we have survived a flood. This book is not about living the "right" life, surviving cancer the "right" way. It is about finding our own way. For some of us, having had cancer means that we don't have time to waste; for others of us, it means that wasting time is our greatest luxury. For some, it means pushing to achieve our ambitions; for others, it means releasing ourselves from worldly ambition. As life goes on, we each sort out what it means to be a survivor.

Some changes begin immediately after our diagnosis, as we decide what is important and weed out those things that we think waste our time. Deeper changes, however, only come with time. It takes several years to move through the phases of limbo that are discussed here—disorientation, fears of recurrence and a preoccupation with death, and grief and an abiding awareness of loss. As we work through these feelings, we understand what has happened to us in ever-changing ways. Lisa read a particular article on survival several months after her treatment and thought it was "okay." Two years later, she found the same article a brilliant debriefing of life after cancer. Certain things don't make sense until we have had time to absorb them.

That is what this chapter is about. Dancing in limbo is the last and longest phase of surviving; it is when we find our own way and make sense of life. I had hoped that Lisa and I could write this final chapter together. She had to remind me that she has no stories to tell because she isn't at this phase yet. Even though she had made her life more satisfying in many ways, she does not yet have the full perspective. She is still grieving many losses and cannot be in a place she hasn't come to yet. That is true for all of us.

Telling Time

Most cancer survivors tell time by their cancer: there is "before" and "after" cancer. This way of marking time suggests the magnitude of the event. As many survivors have noted, cancer changes everything. Shelley Taylor found that cancer patients consistently describe a discontinuity in time before and after their diagnosis and treatment. She believes that patients need to emphasize the difference in their lives in order to believe that the cancer will not come back, to believe that since things are so different now, the cancer will not happen again. Bente, for example, clearly articulated this belief.

I think the break in time goes deeper. It is a break in our experience of ourselves. Like Humpty Dumpty after the fall, we cannot put ourselves back together in the old way. Remember that it took both time and the help of a good therapist for Ellen to figure this out: "I had changed, and I had kept thinking that I would go back to exactly who I was before having the melanoma." We can never go back to who we were before. We know too much about ourselves and the world.

The core of the difference in my life before and after cancer is captured in a dream I had several days before I went to the dentist about the sore in my mouth. In the dream, nothing happened, and everything changed. It was dusk, and there was a large spreading oak tree. An old woman sat with her legs crossed on one of the lower branches. She had a beautifully wrinkled face and flowing gray hair. Her bare feet dangled beneath a long skirt. I was drawn to her, and as she looked at me, I knew she was my death, sitting in that tree. I woke, and with no sense of alarm, I believed that I had cancer.

For me, that dream is not only my first meeting with death, it is the essence of limbo: nothing obvious is happening and everything has changed. I have met my death. She is no one else's. Having seen her, I cannot forget.

I tell this story reluctantly because I do not want to be misunderstood. I do not believe that dreams foretell the future. However, I do believe in the unconscious and the human imagination. Our dreams express both. My dream embodied my unconscious sense that a sore in my mouth that would not heal was not benign.

As in my dream, after cancer we know that we are mortal and the world is not benign. Not only can bad things happen to good people, something bad has already happened to us. We are both shaken by this knowledge and set free. On the day that I was diagnosed, I wrote in my journal:

> If I survive this, and that is a BIG IF, I promise to take more risks and to realize who I can be. Enough of being afraid and holding myself back. There is a wonderful perspective in all of this, which is not detachment but a clarity about what matters and what does not. I want to hold on to this clarity and courage—a funny word because I suddenly understand it so differently, not like brave and daring. The courage to take risks comes down to knowing what matters and doing it, for the simple reason that it matters, and most of my fears do not.

A new world is open to us. It is a more frightening place, but it is real, and in it we can risk being ourselves. When we really get it that we are going to die, along with fear, many of us experience a dizzying freedom. Bente vividly remembered her initial reaction to the diagnosis of invasive cervical cancer. She literally ran—out of her house and into a neighboring field. She was running away, running to exhaust her terror. When she collapsed, panting, she began to laugh. No matter how hard she ran, she could not get away from herself. Maybe it was time to reevaluate her life. The long, slow process of reclaiming more of herself began that day. As she characterized it, "A particular unraveling of my personal history came with my cancer. Ultimately, I found freedom in the experience." Out of her newfound freedom, Bente made important changes in her life.

Revising Our Lives

Surviving a life-threatening illness frequently prompts a reevaluation of life. Those who care for the dying have observed the phenomenon of life review. If people have the time, energy, and courage as they face death, they evaluate their lives. In that summing up, both what they have done *and* what they leave undone is counted. Survivors are thrown into a similar process.

Over half of the cancer patients interviewed by Taylor's group reported that the cancer experience had caused them to reappraise their lives. The survivors Lisa and I talked to began by asking, Why me? Will I live or die? But those questions gave way to deeper questions of existence: Why am I here? How do I want to live my life?

Shortly after her surgery, Lisa took what all of us who loved her thought was a big risk. As she remembers it:

> I decided to go ahead and move to the country. I bought a house that needed some work, but it was what I'd always really wanted. Being in a peaceful place away from cities was more important to me than ever before. I found the place three months after my surgery. My friends said, "Don't do it. Save your money and energy to get well." I felt deep down that I needed this house, as a symbol of hope that I'd live to enjoy it, and because it was a statement about how I wanted to live my life—close to nature, with quiet and beauty.

The death threat becomes the catalyst for restructuring our lives along more meaningful lines. As Judy put it, "Cancer gets your attention. You begin to focus on what's really important to you." Thus begins the creation of an authentic life. For Lisa and me and for the survivors we met, the meaning of life is a pressing issue, but it is not a grand abstraction. It comes down to a deceptively simple thing—how we spend our time.

Dorothy, as we have seen, came to understand the link between meaning and time through her image of her life as "a variety of concentric circles" spreading outward. She found she had been spending time on the "outer ring," but after her diagnosis and treatment, she tried to spend her time with the "rings that are much closer in and more significant."

The task is straightforward. First, we must determine what is truly important to us. Then we must commit our time and energy to it. Jeannette, nearing eighty, had survived the death of her daughter and her husband, as well as her own lung cancer. Describing her revised philosophy of life, she said, "You don't have time to waste. Whatever you want to do, do it. When you're alive and well and kicking. . . . Don't wait. I mean, it's not like . . . you're immortal." Every survivor knew the task, and each confessed that it was more easily said than done.

Creating Meaning

Creating our own lives takes courage. We will probably disappoint ourselves and others. First, we will disappoint by saying no to all the things we cannot see and do and be. In order to focus and commit, we must recognize and accept our limits—time, energy, money. Despite the advertising campaign, we cannot have it all, and that is a disappointment to the greedy grandiose child in us all. But second, and far more frightening, is the possibility that we may choose, commit, and fail. We could fall flat on our faces. Barbara used skating as a metaphor for life as she talked about the possibility of failing: "I decided that I don't want to be afraid of life anymore. Sometimes you hold yourself back. . . . You don't want to go too fast when you're skating because you're afraid you might fall. Or you don't even want to skate because you're afraid you might hurt yourself. . . . I just want to embrace things. I want to do them because we don't really know how long we have."

Another survivor described his cancer experience as an "early midlife crisis." Neil was thirty-two when he was diagnosed with testicular cancer twenty years ago. Although the prospects for a cure are quite good today, back then he faced almost certain death. Neil fought for his chemotherapy and became one of the early successes in the treatment of testicular cancer. When faced with death, he took charge of his life. As he tells it, "At thirty-two, I woke up to the fact that I'm going to die, and . . . I don't want to waste my time. So you recognize that your time is limited and precious, and that you . . . have some control over it." As in a midlife crisis, Neil's reordering of priorities turned his life upside down. But in the new order, he found a sense of meaning and purpose.

Recreating our lives on new terms allows us to go on. These terms can include not only our own death but anything from a physical handicap to an abandoned relationship or career. Martina had been a successful attorney with a busy private practice when she took time out to deliver her first child. She was diagnosed with non-Hodgkin's lymphoma when her son was three months old and underwent a rigorous course of chemotherapy. She never resumed her law practice. "Nothing has ever been the same since I had cancer," she says. The disease became the catalyst for a major life change. Looking back, she says, "I can't imagine how I would have got my life together any other way. I was definitely on the wrong track, full-speed ahead, and not happy. It would have taken a pretty big crisis to get me to open my eyes." Martina didn't change her life in the hope of averting a recurrence. Rather, the crisis of cancer became an opportunity for her to create a new and more satisfying life.

Ellen tells a similar story. She lost her marriage but came to view that loss as a positive change in her life. In listening to Ellen, it is immediately clear that she places great value on her relationships. She describes the diagnosis and treatment of her melanoma in terms of its effect on her parents, friends, and husband. A year and a half after her skin cancer was treated, she developed a suspicious lump in her breast. At that time, her husband left her. As she relates this sequence of events, she does not cast herself as a victim. Instead, she explains that her marriage had begun to unravel with her melanoma: "It was really the catalyst for me [to say], 'I'm dissatisfied in this marriage. Life is short. I want to live.'" She assumed responsibility for the state of her marriage and her life. First, she tried to make the marriage work, but when her efforts failed and her husband left, Ellen got on with her life. Her illusions about her marriage were shattered, but with the help of a caring therapist, she learned that she is "far more resilient" than she had known. Twelve years later, her story is not about cancer; it is about her ongoing search for "what life's all about."

When survivors speak of their lives "before" and "after" cancer, they are acknowledging the major life changes precipitated by the crisis. For some survivors, the visible structure of their lives is not dramatically changed, but they feel completely different on the inside. Judy reported that her experience with breast cancer brought focus to her life: "I was kind of floundering before. My life is not so much different now, but it sure feels different." For Dorothy, the changes were also more internal than external. As she described the basic shift in emphasis in her life since her bout with breast cancer, she noted: "I've been doing some reading and [I] hear people who have completely changed their lives, and I think, 'I don't really want to change my life.' Actually, I like my life."

My own response was much like Dorothy's: my strongest sense in the first year after my cancer was not only how much I wanted to live but also how much I loved my life. I did not want to make any external changes. I wanted to stop struggling within myself to be someone other than me. An image formed in my mind. I was of the earth. Before cancer, I had been sedimentary rock. Fossils, leafprints, watermarks—the accumulated experiences of my life—were embedded in my layers. After cancer, I was metamorphic rock. Transformed by the intensity of the experience, I had become marble.

That image proved more accurate than I knew. It both captured a change that defied words, and it comforted me. I was solid. I was profoundly different and still the same. The raw material had always been there in me. Under pressure, I had taken a stronger form. I did not yet know that surviving would take all my newfound strength and more.

We Fought for Our Lives

One of the major differences in our lives before and after cancer is that after cancer we know that we have fought for our lives and that we have probably sacrificed a part of our body to

the cause. With birth, life is simply given to us; we didn't ask
for it. Cancer threatens to take that life away, and it is no idle
threat. Afterward, we can never take life for granted again. The
effect is profound. Barbara remembered that when she was
most afraid that she would die, she cried because she knew that
she was not ready to go. "It makes you appreciate things more.
Would I see another sunrise? Would I see another flower bloom
in spring? It got a little maudlin, and I thought, 'God, this is
so corny; it would play badly in a theater.' But you go through
those very thoughts." Remember how simply Judy said it, "I
had to keep my focus. I wanted to live. That's what made it
worth sacrificing my breast." Both Barbara and Judy felt a
tremendous loss with their mastectomies. But the choice was
clear, they wanted to live.

   Norm's story is more complicated. As he sees it, he had
always had a self-destructive streak and periods of depression,
even before his melanoma was diagnosed five years ago. When
a friend committed suicide, Norm remembers viewing his
friend's body at the funeral: "He was lying there in the casket,
and I was jealous. I envied him. He was done. . . . At that point
in time, there was a big part of me that wanted to die. Life was
too hard. I wanted out." Then his melanoma was diagnosed.
Death was a real possibility. Late at night, in his hospital room,
Norm talked it over with his god. He reached a state of peace.
"[I said], 'If it's my time to go right now, I'm ready.' And yet
I also said that 'I don't want to go.' I made a request, and that
was very freeing for me. It changed my outlook and my life."
For perhaps the first time, Norm made a commitment to him-
self and to life.

> My life changed when I said that I didn't want to go. Some-
> thing shifted in me, and very, very, very slowly I started to
> make decisions and changes in my life that would make my life
> more pleasant and make things more attractive to me to want
> to stick around. This wasn't a quest. It just sort of started hap-
> pening. I got plugged back into some real nurturing friends.
> I was in therapy, and I turned that up a notch. I started a very

slow process of separating from my wife. [They subsequently divorced.] I'm still in the change mode, and it's been five years.

We may not want to identify with Norm's self-destructive streak, but most of us have felt at times that life is too hard. If we are rock-bottom honest, most of us want life to be simpler and easier. We want more things to go our way. When we face death and say, "No, not yet, please. I want to live some more," we are accepting life as it is. We are not saying, "I only want to live if it will be happily ever after." We want to be alive, period. We recognize that life may be more difficult if we survive. That is acceptable. We will lose our hair, sacrifice our breasts; we will do whatever it takes.

Among survivors, there is often a large measure of acceptance of what has been, because it has never been ideal. Ellen faced the fact that her marriage was not working. Judy could talk about floundering, Martina of being on the wrong track. They spoke without shame. It was simply the truth as they saw it, and they recognized an opportunity to do things differently with the rest of their lives.

For me, the greatest challenge has always been accepting myself. My life had been very good, but I had never been a good enough girl. I fell painfully short of the standards of grace and decorum that had been prescribed for me. Somehow cancer freed me to doubt the standard instead of always doubting myself. The change was immediate. I had not yet had the biopsy, but I knew that I had cancer. An hour earlier, my dentist had seen the lesion. As I drove from his office to my husband's office, my life did not pass before my eyes. I saw the gray Dallas skyline and superimposed on the tall buildings, each of my major sins stared back at me. They were no longer monstrous, they were my baby steps. They were the handful of times that I had trusted my intuition and broken with the rules. In the awkward struggle to find myself, I had hurt others—my parents and my ex-husband, to be sure. I could not undo the harm, but for the first time, I saw that each of my clumsy acts had brought me closer to who I was that day. For the first time, all of me was acceptable to me. I was a mixed bag, just like everyone else.

In addition to accepting ourselves as we are and life as it is, we accept responsibility for the quality of the life we choose. Both Martina and Judy took active steps to improve the quality of their lives. When Martina thought about the major changes she had made in her life, cancer took on a different meaning: "I don't feel like it was a horrible experience. At a physical level it was gruesome, but that . . . wasn't the important part." The important part was creating a life that satisfied her soul. Judy felt physically deformed by the loss of her breast, "I felt a lot of sadness in the first year. I was walking around with no breast. I really didn't like that. I'd lost a very important part of my body—a part I was really fond of." After she had grieved the loss, she had her breast reconstructed. Now she feels whole again and deeply changed. Much like Martina, Judy acknowledges the misery of having cancer while also valuing the changes in her life, "Cancer is a nightmare. It's horrible. And it can have incredibly positive aspects. It is life-changing in the best sense."

Time on Our Side

Maintaining the quality of our lives requires constant vigilance. Remembering that we are going to die actually helps us with the task. Most of the survivors Lisa and I met were acutely aware of time. They not only divided their lives into the time before and after cancer, they were especially mindful of how they spent their time. Nearly everyone said, in one way or another, "I don't have time to waste." Judy said it concisely, "I have a heightened sense of not wasting time. Not wasting my life." Ann had concluded: "I don't have time to fool around. If I don't want to do something, I won't do it. I think that change has to do with the cancer. Life is too short to do things you don't want to do anymore." One of the things she wanted to do was relax: "I love to waste time now." Since time is our most precious possession, wasting it is the greatest luxury.

Neil was acutely aware of how easily he could drift off course: "The clarity has clearly slipped away at times." "In the first month or so," he remembered, "I was very clear, and the only thing I was focusing on was living. Was I going to be here joyfully or not? I wasn't worried about money. I wasn't worried about my relationship. I wasn't worried about the future. I was focused on this moment and how I was spending it. It didn't have to be puritanism where I was always being productive. Peace of mind and living in the moment and living these moments in life, these seconds, that was the only priority." None of us can maintain such intensity, but we want to hold onto a piece of it, and even that isn't always easy. Martina knew this: "There's something to draw from my cancer experience, but I have to take time enough to relax and . . . tune into it. Sometimes it takes a minor kick in the butt to do it."

Virginia brings a special perspective to the meaning of time. While the cancer she had early in her life prompted one set of changes, the serious scare of a recurrence that she had in her mid fifties, prompted another: "I've made a very conscious decision to change my life completely. When I first had cancer, one of the by-products was a drivenness . . . to maximize every single moment and to do something with it. What I've now decided is to take time out to do something differently every day, even if it's something small. I'll wake up in the morning and say, 'Okay, what is it that I'm going to do differently today?' And I know that with that attitude, something different will occur because I'm more attentive, more focused."

Most survivors appeared to value quiet time, especially time alone with themselves, more than they had before. Dorothy's comment was typical: "I choose to spend my time more carefully and also to take more time for reflection." Developing an inner life, a life of the soul, emerged as a theme. Martina observed: "There are times when I get off track . . . and don't do the thing that satisfies my soul. I sort of wander off and pull myself back and wander off and pull myself back." The question Judy "regularly" asked herself was, "What am I doing here in this lifetime?" Each survivor has developed the ability to call herself or himself to account.

Spiritual Questions

Many of the survivors talked about finding a spiritual force in their lives. They did not use the shared language of religious traditions, although some of them are members of traditional religious faiths. They spoke in a personal language from their direct experience. Judy noted, "Cancer thrust me into a much more conscious spiritual quest, for lack of better words." Martina characterized her cancer as a "spiritual crisis," emphasizing that "I definitely have a spiritual life now and a spiritual perspective that I never had before." Dorothy said, "I've gotten into meditation and just developing a spiritual side, which I hadn't done before. And actually it's a wonderful experience." The survivors' focus is on enriching the quality of their lives today. As Judy said, "It's a constant process of deepening my understanding of life."

Several of the survivors raised the question of an afterlife. Brian was thirty-four when his melanoma was diagnosed. After years of drifting, he had finally settled down, creating a happy marriage with two young sons and a promising career as a scientist. This was no time to die. For Brian, his potentially fatal disease raised not only "all of the issues around mortality" but also questions about "the transition to whatever, if anything, lies ahead." With considerable wit, he described himself as "a thinking man, a person who has never known or loved a god, and who cannot count on divine intervention in times of personal crisis." Brian was on his own, and he knew it, "I carry with me no sense of religious specialness to lend strength in the face of danger. In fact, I have never had much natural faith that things will turn out for the best under any circumstances." Given his natural skepticism, Brian finds life most satisfying when he stops worrying and just lives, and the most useful answers come from heartfelt experience, not the logic of his fine mind. Brian has found both strength and inspiration in the courage of others. His careful attention to the dying members of his cancer support group is both a gift of love to them and a gift to himself. Through them, he is learning how to die. He hopes that he won't need to use the lessons anytime soon, but he is grateful all the same.

For Bill, however, facing death prompted a leap of faith. "I decided that there was some form of existence after the death of the body. It was really obvious to me. . . . Until I had that confrontation with death, it wasn't something that I needed to know." Remember that Bill is an accomplished artist who painted throughout his radiation treatments. One of the scenes from that period is a "woman having a vision of life after death." In his current work, images of portals appear, which he describes as "gateways to another life." That visual metaphor is reminiscent of Bente's verbal image of cancer as "a major doorway." Bill is quick to argue that such paintings are not necessarily a "response to having had cancer"; however, death has found a way into his work.

Bill's spiritual awakening was an epiphany, but such dramatic shifts were rare. Most of the people Lisa and I talked with either felt their existing faith deepen or embarked upon a gradual course of spiritual self-discovery. Virginia has had three brushes with death and years to struggle with "the meaning of life and the meaning of dying." Now in her early fifties, she reports, "It's been a slow process. I went from being an agnostic to being a gnostic, and I don't know when. But I have no doubt now. It's a knowingness. It's not a faith, not a belief system. It's occurred in the last couple of years. I know it's not complete, because whenever cancer comes up and the fear, I clutch . . . and there isn't that greater-beingness. This is a whole new territory for me." The world of the spirit may be new territory, but these survivors are also explorers. They did not discuss their evolving spirituality as if they had found religion in the face of death. They were not doing what it might take to gain admission to an afterlife. They were developing a neglected aspect of themselves to enrich their lives now, and their spirituality was very much a work in progress.

Giving Each Other Courage

I came a long way in the short drive from my dentist's office, when my sins were not as large as skyscrapers, but the journey had just begun. Diagnosis and treatment were not the hardest parts for me. Hard as they were, and surely time has faded their darkest moments, surviving has been harder—living with fear and loss, living with my own wounds and, therefore, sensitized to the raw places in others. The crisis passes; these things endure.

I grow less confident of my rightness with every year. Perhaps that is because I was so cocksure in the extended adolescence of my young adult years, when I knew the truth about damn near everything. That brand of confidence is gone. I am a middle-aged woman with a warm smile and sad eyes. I was able to do my part of writing this book precisely because I know that I do not have the answers. I do know that cancer was part of finding myself. But it has not been all of the story. My analysis, my mother's death, my aging body, the deaths of friends, all of those have brought me to who I am today.

None of the survivors believed that he or she had "the answer," but each was asking important questions. Judy said of life that "all we can do is get an idea of how it works for us. I'm suspicious of anyone who claims to have answers." Unlike Oscar Wilde's character in *Lady Windermere's Fan* who cautions that "life is far too important a thing to ever talk seriously about," these survivors talked about serious and sacred things. They were earnest and funny, articulate and at a loss for words. Virginia seemed to sum it up: "I want to be less stuffy about important issues. I've taken myself too seriously, and I don't want to anymore. Life is just too short."

Clearly, the survivors spoke from their souls. Many of them revealed the most intimate details of their illnesses and their lives. In part, they trusted Lisa and me because we are also survivors. But they didn't know us. They talked to strangers in the hope that their experiences would be useful to other survivors. They told their stories with humility. As Brian said, "I would not be so bold as to try to teach others about cancer survival. I'm merely trying to survive myself."

Socorro had learned the hard way that her coping style did not work for everyone. In fact, respecting the differences between herself and others had been a valuable lesson:

> I have to learn that people deal with things in their own way. I had a friend who called [when she found out she had cancer], and I said, "Wait. I'll drive over with my cardboard box [full of books on cancer] and my files." And she said, "Why?" And I said, "Don't you want to read about it? Don't you want to know what to ask the doctor? Don't you want to make a list of questions?" And she said, "No." I was just so taken aback. But it made me realize that there's more than one way to skin a cat.

Just as we and the other survivors each dealt with our cancer in our own way, now all of us survive in our own ways. Our revised lives take many forms, but there are common features: self-respect, trusting our intuition, finding the understanding, support, and love we need, taking responsibility for the quality of our lives, and risking commitment to what truly matters to us. Virginia spoke for many of us when she said, "I try to have a lot more self-acceptance and forgiveness."

When asked what he would say to other cancer survivors, Norm wasn't bashful: "You are the only you you've got. You're special, and whatever it takes to reclaim some love for yourself or whatever you need to do to start making moves and decisions that will feel good for you . . . get on that track, and things will progressively get better. It sounds clichéd, but it's my truth."

It is a curious thing that as I end this book, my memories circle back to the beginning of my time with cancer. During the week before I was diagnosed, when I had a sense of what was coming, I found a dragonfly in a gutter. Its delicate wings were perfectly intact, as was the body with its long, slender segments. As I gently lifted the dead insect and cupped it in the palm of my left hand, I told Curtis about my childhood wish to fly.

When I was four, I wanted three things with desperation. I wanted to read, to swim, and to fly. I pretended to do all three. I held the daily paper before my eyes and made the muttering sounds my father made as he scanned the news. I lay belly down in my play pool with my head arched up out of the water, one arm beneath me, supporting myself with a sly hand on the plastic floor: "Mommy, I can swim." She would smile and nod and never call my bluff. Before long, she had taught me to read and arranged for swimming lessons. Dreams were coming true, but flight continued to elude me.

By the time I was seven, I had resorted to lying about my flights. For my attempts, I would put on my filmiest nightgown, like the one worn by the elfin girls with dragonfly wings in one of my storybooks. One day, my father left a ladder against the grape arbor in our backyard after he had been working there. I climbed up and surveyed the yard and our neighbor's yard. I could see a lot from up there. Then I jumped. It was not the landing of my dreams, but I ran right in to announce another successful flight. The ladder disappeared. However, I knew where there was a stepstool. So I took to carrying the stool into the yard after school to practice my technique. I would come home, change into my nightgown, and go to work.

It had to be spring and I had to be seven because my brother, Eddy, was four. He had announced that he was going to be an alligator when he grew up, and the neighborhood boys had called him a liar. He fought for his honor and the pride of all alligators and came home with a bloody nose. I was considering my own career options, and I wanted something that guaranteed flight. Usually, I planned to be a bird. I would lie on my back in the grass and watch birds soar overhead. I just knew that I could do it. Then the air turned to butterflies, huge monarchs. Within several years, the DDT used throughout California's central valley would wipe them out. But that year, there were still masses of them, and I reconsidered my future.

I did what I always did when considering important life matters. I got out my *World Book Encyclopedia* to look up what I wanted to know: in this case, butterflies. I read about the larva and the pupa. Then I got to the part about the winged adult—it lived for seventeen days. At least, that's how I remember it. Seventeen days was far too short a life span. Butterflies were out. All this drifted through me as I stood on a street curb with a dead dragonfly in my hand, suspecting that I had cancer.

I felt deeply connected to the stubbornly imaginative little girl I had once been, and I wanted her to live. There had been a time when I had refused to have my hopes and dreams thwarted by harsher realities. I was about to face such a time again. I needed my little girl and her wish to fly. The core of my will to live was, and still is, embodied in that child and the adult in me who protects her.

Life and Death and Limbo

When I was lost in limbo, I felt utterly alone. No one seemed to have been there before me, so I had no guide. The saddest thing about my first years in limbo is how hard I worked to live the myth that nothing had really changed. I tried to make my survival a nonevent. Surviving cancer *is* a big deal: a big, wonderful, horrible, important, mundane, crazy, sad, and joyous long-running event.

At the end of her interview, Judy said: "There are many ways in which I consider cancer a great gift. There's no PR on the subject, and it's a complicated concept to get across." That complicated concept is exactly what we have hoped to communicate. We have told the truth of our lives in limbo because forgetting the truth of survival has a terrible cost: all of us lose our connection to who we are and how we feel.

There is a wonderful country and western song called "The Dance." It is, of course, a brokenhearted love song, but the last lines are as appropriate to surviving cancer as they are to surviving a lost love:

Life is better left to chance.
I could have missed the pain,
But I'd . . . have missed the dance.

In the middle of writing this book, I watched my mother die—a slow, miserable death. Her dying broke my heart. However, with this heartbreak, I knew that the pain truly was part of the dance. And ultimately, I was able to mend my broken heart with grief and gratitude for all the people I love who love me back—even when I lose them.

Throughout my time with cancer, I needed other people's love and confidence in me because my own had been shaken. I needed the image of my mother and grandmother who had survived cancer before me. I learned to heal myself by surviving cancer. I learned that illness and injury and sadness and death are not my enemies. They are essential parts of life.

Limbo is a place inside ourselves, and therefore not a place at all: it is a paradox. It is neither heaven nor hell, and there is no way out. There is only waiting, and as we wait, we wonder: Will I live or will I die? At first the question is specific. We are thinking about our cancer. Then we realize the absurdity of our question. Of course, we are going to die. That realization is not abstract. It is a swirling in our belly and a buzzing in our head. It is the human condition: to live in the full knowledge of our own inevitable death.

In our lives after cancer, we are learning to dance with life and death: we are alive *and* we are mortal. The dance in limbo requires all our strength and flexibility, but it also requires balance. Through the dance, we express ourselves and we communicate with others—soul to soul. Expression and connection—that is what dancing in limbo is all about.

Resources

Further Reading

There are a great many books about cancer: first-person accounts, self-help books on treatment and prevention issues, cooking and diet suggestions, and so forth. Although some of the books we have listed here are directly concerned with cancer, others are not. Our object was to list those resources that offered us insights into the territory of limbo and helped us in learning the steps necessary to dance in that territory.

Becker, E. *The Denial of Death*. New York: Free Press, 1973.
In this dense and brilliant book about the human need to deny the presence of death, Becker argues that our repression of the knowledge of our own death is the source of much of our behavior and the basis for anxiety. The preface and chapters one through four are especially recommended.

Carter, R., with Galant, S. *Helping Yourself Help Others: A Book for Caregivers*. New York: Times Books, 1994.
Although the emphasis in this book is on the care of the elderly, the treatment of caregiver issues is thorough and thoughtful. The book is written for the general public rather than professional caregivers and is consequently very readable.

Fiore, N. A. *The Road Back to Health: Coping with the Emotional Aspects of Cancer*. Berkeley, Calif.: Celestial Arts, 1990.
This practical guide to living with cancer from the time of diagnosis, written by a psychotherapist who is a cancer survivor, emphasizes the psychological and emotional skills for coping with and communicating about cancer.

161

Healing and the Mind, with Bill Moyers. New York: Doubleday, 1993. Based on the public television series of the same name, *Healing and the Mind* explores the relationship between mind and body and looks at healing approaches that are outside Western medicine. The section "Wounded Healers" interviews people at the Commonweal Cancer Help Program in Bolinas, California.

Horowitz, K. E., and Lanes, D. M. *Witness to Illness: Strategies for Caregiving and Coping.* Reading, Mass.: Addison-Wesley, 1992. This personal and compelling account of one caregiver's experience takes you into the issues confronting "witnesses" to serious illness and offers understanding and advice to people who are in that role.

Kalish, R. A. *Death, Grief, and Caring Relationships.* Pacific Grove, Calif.: Brooks/Cole, 1981. This scholarly and easy-to-read text on death and dying discusses the meaning of death, the process of dying, grief and bereavement, and the health and mental health professionals involved in these processes.

Le Shan, L. *Cancer as a Turning Point: A Handbook for People with Cancer, Their Families and Health Professionals.* New York: Dutton, 1989. Psychotherapist Le Shan summarizes mind-body and immune system research and discusses his belief that cancer can be a turning point for creating meaning in our lives, so we are "glad to get up in the morning and glad to go to bed at night."

Nessim, S., and Ellis, J. *Cancervive: The Challenge of Life After Cancer.* Boston: Houghton Mifflin, 1991. Nessim and Ellis emphasize some of the practical aspects of surviving cancer, such as job rights and obtaining health insurance. Nessim is cofounder of Cancervive, a national support group.

Mullan, F., Hoffman, B., and the Editors of Consumer Reports Books. *Charting the Journey: An Almanac of Practical Resources for Cancer Survivors.* Mount Vernon, N.Y.: Consumers Union, 1990. This reference work contains practical information as well as articles about emotional issues affecting survivors. It has an extensive annotated section of national resource organizations.

Price, R. *A Whole New Life: An Illness and a Healing.* New York: Atheneum, 1994. An eloquent, thoughtful, and honest personal account of surviving spinal cancer, written by one of America's finest living authors and bringing a distinctly male perspective to the experience of survival.

Rinpoche, S. *The Tibetan Book of Living and Dying.* San Francisco: HarperSanFrancisco, 1992.

Buddhist meditation master Rinpoche teaches the Tibetan perspective of life and death and the belief that we can go beyond denial and fear of death to discover what is central and changeless in ourselves.

Spiegel, D. *Living Beyond Limits: New Hope and Help for Facing Life-Threatening Illness.* New York: Random House, 1993.
A readable and compassionate book based on research by the author and others at Stanford University. The research found that women with metastatic breast cancer who attended a support group significantly improved the quality of their lives and also lived twice as long as women who did not attend a group.

Vaillant, G. *Adaptation to Life.* Boston: Little, Brown, 1977.
This is a classic work on psychological defenses. Written for a general reading audience, the book makes these often difficult concepts understandable through the use of numerous examples from the everyday lives of a large group of men.

Viorst, J. *Necessary Losses: The Loves, Illusions, Dependencies, and Impossible Expectations That All of Us Have to Give Up in Order to Grow.* New York: Simon & Schuster, 1986.
Viorst's thesis is that loss is part of life and that the way we deal with loss is central to our personal growth and understanding of ourselves. Chapters cover losses of childhood, of impossible expectations in relationships, of our own younger selves, and of people we love.

Wilber, K. *Grace and Grit: Spirituality and Healing in the Life and Death of Treya Killam Wilber.* Boston: Shambhala, 1993.
Ken Wilber weaves together his journals and those of his wife during the years of her battle with breast cancer. This human experience changed Wilber's theoretical New Age belief system, and he discusses his evolution throughout the book.

Yalom, I. D. *Existential Psychotherapy.* New York: Basic Books, 1980.
This definitive text on existential psychology provides a clear, elegant explanation of the complex ways in which people deal with the important issues of existence: meaning, isolation, freedom, and death anxiety.

Helpful Organizations

The following organizations can help you locate information about specific kinds of cancer and about a variety of self-help and support groups. We have listed only national organizations. They can give you information about your regional and local groups when appropriate.

American Cancer Society, 1599 Clifton Road N.E., Atlanta, GA 30329; (800) ACS-2345 (for national and local information).
The American Cancer Society (ACS) is an information and referral service providing general information on prevention, diagnosis, research, treatment, support, publications, and ACS itself. ACS also sponsors several grass-roots cancer support programs (contact your local ACS unit for information about the support programs in your area):

> *CanSurmount* brings together survivors, family members, survivor volunteers, and health professionals to provide mutual support and education.

> *I Can Cope* addresses the educational and psychological needs of survivors and family members through a series of eight classes.

> *Reach to Recovery* provides rehabilitation support for women who have had breast cancer. It makes hospital visits and supplies temporary prostheses.

American Self-Help Clearinghouse, St. Clare's–Riverside Medical Center, 25 Pocono Road, Denville, NJ 07834; (201) 625–7101; (800) FOR-MASH (356–6274), New Jersey only.
This clearinghouse helps people locate resources about many health issues including cancer. It also publishes *The Self-Help Sourcebook: Finding and Forming Mutual Aid Self-Help Groups,* which lists over five hundred national self-help groups by name and contact address.

Living with Cancer Self-Help Group, Better Health and Medical Forum, America Online.
This electronic forum meets on Sundays at 7:00 P.M. ET.

Make Today Count, St. John's Regional Health Center, 1235 E. Cherokee, Springfield, MO 65804; (800) 432–2273.
Make Today Count is a national organization of more than two hundred chapters that provide emotional self-help to survivors and their families. Chapter activities include formal programs, group discussions, newsletters, social events, workshops and seminars, and educational programs.

National Alliance of Breast Cancer Organizations, 1180 Avenue of the Americas (2nd floor), New York, NY 10036; (212) 719–0154.
This is a clearinghouse for breast cancer information and organizations.

National Cancer Institute, Cancer Information Service, Building 31, Room 10A16, Bethesda, MD 20892; (800) 4-CANCER (422–6237); in Alaska, call (800) 638–1234.
This service answers questions about cancer and offers a wide variety of free consumer publications about cancer prevention, diagnosis, and treatment. It also operates Physician Data Query (PDQ), which pro-

vides information about treatment, including the most current results from investigational trials. Spanish-speaking staff members are available to callers from certain areas.

National Coalition for Cancer Survivorship, 1010 Wayne Avenue (5th floor), Silver Spring, MD 20910; (301) 650–8868.
The coalition, founded in 1986, is a clearinghouse for information on survivorship, including nationwide support groups, insurance and employment issues, and advocacy for cancer survivors. The coalition can assist individuals in starting cancer support and networking systems. It also publishes a newsletter and sponsors survivorship conferences.

National Self-Help Clearinghouse, City University of New York, Graduate School and University Center, 25 West Forty-Third Street, Room 620, New York, NY 10036; (212) 354–8525.
This clearinghouse supplies cancer self-help resources as well as information on many other topics. Call for information about support groups in your area.

Chapter References

Epigraph

Milton, J. *Paradise Lost,* 3:498 (1667).

Chapter One

American Cancer Society. *Cancer Facts and Figures, 1994.* Atlanta: American Cancer Society, 1994.

Chapter Two

Dunkel-Schetter, C., Feinstein, L., Taylor, S., and Falke, R. "Patterns of Coping with Breast Cancer." *Health Psychology,* 1992, *11*(2), 79–87.

Kaysen, S. *Girl, Interrupted.* New York: Turtle Bay Books, 1993, p. 42.

Koopman, C., Classen, C., and Spiegel, D. "Predictors of Posttraumatic Stress Symptoms Among Survivors of the Oakland/Berkeley, Calif., Firestorm." *American Journal of Psychiatry,* 1994, *151*(6), 888–894.

Chapter Three

Bearison, D. J., Sadow, A. J., Granowetter, L., Winkel, G. "Patients' and Parents' Causal Attributions for Childhood Cancer." *Journal of Psychosocial Oncology,* 1993, *11,* 47–61.

Holland, J. Personal communication, Feb. 27, 1995.

Price, R. *A Whole New Life: An Illness and a Healing.* New York: Atheneum, 1994, p. 53.

Taylor, S. "Adjustment to Threatening Events: A Theory of Cognitive Adaptation." *American Psychologist,* 1983, *38*(11), 1161–1173.

Williams, T. "Diagnosis and Treatment of Survivor Guilt." In J. P. Wilson, Z. Harel, and B. Kahana (eds.), *Human Adaptation to Extreme Stress: From the Holocaust to Vietnam.* New York: Plenum, 1988, pp. 319–336.

Chapter Four

Lamott, A. *Bird by Bird: Some Instructions on Writing and Life.* New York: Pantheon Books, 1994, p. 146.

Spiegel, D. *Living Beyond Limits: New Hope and Help for Facing Life-Threatening Illness.* New York: Random House, 1993.

Chapter Five

Bowlby, J. *Attachment and Loss.* Vol. 3: *Loss: Sadness and Depression.* New York: Basic Books, 1980.

Kalish, R. *Death, Grief, and Caring Relationships.* Pacific Grove, Calif.: Brooks/Cole, 1981.

Parkes, C. *Bereavement: Studies of Grief in Adult Life.* Madison, Conn.: International Universities Press, 1987.

Raphael, B. *The Anatomy of Bereavement.* New York: Basic Books, 1987.

Speca, M., Robinson, J. W., Goodey, E., and Frizell, B. "Patients Evaluate a Quality-of-Life Scale: Whose Life Is It, Anyway?" *Cancer Practice,* 1994, *2*(5), 365–370.

Taylor, S. "Adjustment to Threatening Events: A Theory of Cognitive Adaptation." *American Psychologist,* 1983, *38*(11), 1161–1173.

Chapter Six

Duff, K. *The Alchemy of Illness.* New York: Bell Tower, 1993, p. 39.

Fiore, N. A. *The Road Back to Health: Coping with the Emotional Aspects of Cancer.* Berkeley, Calif.: Celestial Arts, 1990, p. 30.

Houlden, A., Lowery, B. J., and Jacobsen, B. "Self-Blame and Adjustment to Breast Cancer." *Oncology Nursing Forum,* Jan.-Feb. 1996.

Siegel, B. *Peace, Love, and Healing: Bodymind Communication and the Path to Self-Healing: An Exploration.* New York: HarperCollins, 1989, p. 16.

Wilber, K., and Wilber, T. "Do We Make Ourselves Sick?" *New Age Journal,* Sept.-Oct. 1988, p. 51.

Yalom, I. D. *Existential Psychotherapy.* New York: Basic Books, 1980, pp. 274–275.

Chapter Seven

Mishel, M. H., Padilla, G., Grant, M., and Sorenson, D. S. "Uncertainty in Illness Theory: A Replication of the Mediating Effects of Mastery and Coping." *Nursing Research,* 1991, *40*(4), 239.

Waxler-Morrison, N., Hislop, T. G., Mears, B., and Kan, L. "Effects of Social Relationships on Survival for Women with Breast Cancer: A Prospective Study." *Social Science Medicine,* 1991, *33*(2), 177–183.

Chapter Eight

Taylor, S. "Adjustment to Threatening Events: A Theory of Cognitive Adaptation." *American Psychologist,* 1983, *38*(11), 1161–1173.

Acknowledgments

Many people were part of us as we wrote this book. Some participated actively by reading drafts and giving feedback and by sharing their cancer stories. Others were there to love us, give us support, prod us on, and celebrate with us. Still others were important to us when we were sick and recovering. These acknowledgments are our thanks to all of you who made it possible for us to write.

The Other Survivors

Our deep thanks are given to the women and men who talked with us openly and insightfully about their cancer. A few of these individuals were acquaintances before we interviewed them. Most, however, came to us through friends. We now count them as friends. They speak for themselves about their experiences throughout the book.

Norm Armstrong had a melanoma on his arm five years before we interviewed him. He has had no recurrence. Norm is a roofing contractor in his forties.

Nancy Cain had breast cancer one year before our interview. She is in her mid fifties. She and her husband are both retired.

Judy Cash is a fifty-year-old tour consultant who had breast cancer two years ago.

Ann Dragoon-Wasserman is a sixty-year-old physical fitness instructor. She had melanoma on her leg five years before a recurrence in her lymph system. That recurrence was three years before our interview with her.

Charlotte Ferrey is in her forties and had breast cancer three years ago. She had a double mastectomy. Charlotte is a housewife and school board member.

Neil Fiore is a psychologist in his early fifties and the author of *The Road Back to Health: Coping with the Emotional Aspects of Cancer* and other books. Neil had testicular cancer twenty years ago, when testicular cancer was thought always to be fatal.

Bente Friend is a spiritual consultant. She had invasive cervical cancer three years ago, when she was in her late forties.

Dorothy Geoghegan had a single mastectomy for breast cancer two years ago. She is a business consultant in her forties.

Stan Hatch is an attorney in his late fifties. He had breast cancer seven months before our interview, treated with a single mastectomy.

Ellen Jones is an educational consultant who had a melanoma on her leg twelve years ago. Her cancer was discovered before much was known about treating melanoma. She is in her early forties.

Virginia Lewis is a psychotherapist in her early fifties. She had throat cancer thirty years ago.

Socorro Litehiser is an instructional aide in her late forties. She had breast cancer ten years ago and was treated with a single mastectomy.

Bill Martin is an artist, teacher, and writer in his fifties. He had Hodgkin's disease twelve years ago, right after its cure had been discovered.

Martina Reaves had non–Hodgkin's lymphoma eight years ago. She is an attorney who now practices family mediation and pursues art as a hobby. She is in her early forties.

Brian Smith had a melanoma on his back five years ago. He is in his forties and is a geologist and program manager.

Jeannette Waller is a retired professor in her late seventies who had lung cancer four years ago.

Barbara Wayland had breast cancer four years before we met. Three years after her cancer, she had further breast disease, and consequently underwent a double mastectomy with reconstruction. She is a dental hygienist in her early forties.

Katharine Wingbird is a writer in her forties who had cervical cancer a year ago.

Our Mutual Thanks

There are two others to whom we both must give our thanks and appreciation. We want to pay tribute to Richard A. Kalish, a mentor in many senses of the word. Dick was our major professor in graduate school, and it was he who made sure we met each other. His field of study was grief and bereavement, and he taught us both how to study it and live it. Dick died of cancer while we both were writing our dissertations. In our loss of him, our friendship grew. And from that friendship as well as our own experiences with cancer has come this book.

We also want to express affection and appreciation to Becky McGovern, our editor and cheerleader at Jossey-Bass. Becky was with us from the very beginning. She has been a constant source of support and has always been available to help us when our work was difficult and felt overwhelming. Her editorial comments and direction helped give our book its tone and perhaps its soul. Working with Becky has always felt like a three-way collaboration.

Glenna's Thanks

First, I thank Lisa. I neither could nor would have written this book without her. The material was simply too painful to face alone. I have needed to express myself, feel understood, touch others, and "do good" for as long as I can remember. I lived in books as a child, imagining that the people I read about were my friends. I even made my own books of folded paper and sewn seams. I didn't know what to fill them with, so I drew tiny pictures and copied words from real books. Now I have written a real book with my real friend. There are no words in any books to adequately thank you, Lisa.

Other friends kept me on track and saved me from utter loneliness by carefully reading various portions of the manuscript. My thanks to Patricia O'Connor, Kay Monoco, Amy McGrane, Kawana Edwards, Kyle Boyd, Nancy Cain, and Rebel and Chuck Calhoun.

Bea Cunningham was my dream research assistant. Susan Boucher was an always available and wise expert resource. George Peters, M.D., a breast disease specialist, provided insights into cancer treatment and recovery. Joni Mokry, Daniel Barenbaum, and Deidre McCarthy provided valuable information and documents.

Beyond writing there is life. For their loving presence I thank David Metcalf, my analyst, who patiently waited for me to learn to trust him and, thereby, to trust myself; and Mary Ann Shaening, Willa Shalit, and Betty Downes, who were there for me when I could not be there. During Lisa's and my final push to finish the book, Betty reassured me, "Remember, this too shall pass . . . probably like a kidney stone." Thanks.

I also thank my doctors, Jim Williams, John Allen, and Z. H. Lieberman, for each doing their part to save my life. I especially thank Dr. Lieberman for not only saving my life but preserving my ability to speak.

My special thanks to Ed and Roni Halvorson for always being there.

And finally, I have three gratitudes that defy words. First, to my father, Glenn Halvorson, who published his first short story this year, at the age of eighty-one. When he called to tell me the good news, he said, "I beat you to publication." Congratulations, and thank you for being my father. Second, to my mother, Mary Halvorson, who died while I was working on this book. I kept writing as a way to assuage my sense of helplessness in the face of her dying. I also thought writing would be an intellectual distraction, to protect me from the depth of my grief. Instead, the writing forced me to plumb that depth. My mother would have appreciated that irony. Third, and most, to my husband, Curtis Boyd, who decided to take ballroom dancing lessons as I was writing about dancing in limbo. When Curtis proposed to me, he said that he wanted us to grow old together. That is my fondest dream. Now as we grow old, we'll be dancing together.

Lisa's Thanks

I could not have written this book without Glenna. This is obvious on a practical level but also true emotionally. Writing a book about something that mattered to me has been a lifelong dream and therefore full of mental blocks and booby traps. We kept each other steady on the task and spent hours of always satisfying and often painful discussion about life and death. Forming the ideas in the book was like putting together a jigsaw puzzle the size of a living room. Because Glenna has lived in limbo longer than I, she could provide a perspective I do not yet have. I could provide the raw material for many of our concepts, since I was in the middle of fears of recurrence when we began and now am in the grieving phase. I am grateful that we now know that there are new phases of limbo to come, and I am looking forward to the next one, with her as my friend.

So many other friends have given me their love and support—during my cancer, which now seems far away, during the writing of this book, and in my life. In particular, I thank Jane, Emily, Sharon, Betty, Arlin, Mark, Michael, Barbara, Cat, Honey, Simone, and Ellen. They are all ready for me to come and play with them again.

As we celebrate ten years of being in business together, my partner and friend, Donna Lloyd-Kolkin, continues to give me moral support to write as well as her time and energy to cover my projects when I have been immersed in that writing. Thank you.

I appreciate Marilyn White always, this time for keeping me company in the office and for helping with the resources for our book.

Two groups have given me great help. The members of my melanoma support group at UCSF–Mount Zion Cancer Center in San Francisco, led by Andy Kneier, give me a safe place to feel frightened and get comfort. I have learned a lot from those who are ahead of me in life, and I have given back to them what I can. Jan Elliott, Christi Olson, and Anne Karcher allowed me to join their study group for a year to help me meet my writing deadlines.

Steve Walch, my therapist, helps me not to fear my feelings and to believe in my ability to create and sustain loving relationships.

My doctors, Warren Dotz, Michael Cedars, Walter Rohlfing, and David Miller saved my life and gave me beautiful scars.

Although my parents are not alive to witness this realization of my childhood determination to write a book, my three aunts are: Isabella, Ginny, and Martha.

My brother, John, is always there for me. I have known this since he was born, even though we have seldom spoken of the strong bond between us. He is my friend, helper, and architect, and I rely on him more than I know.

And there is always Skip, my magical ally and greatest friend. Our sense of connection is constant, even as we see the world differently: you through the eyes of a painter, sculptor, and craftsman; I through the eyes of a writer.

July 1995   Glenna Halvorson-Boyd, Ph.D.
                               Lisa K. Hunter, Ph.D.
                               Healdsburg, California